Vegan Diet

21 Days of Vegan Recipe Menu Plans and 60+ Recipes

(Vegan Diet to Lose Weight)

Allen Dial

Published by Robert Satterfield Publishing House

© Allen Dial

All Rights Reserved

Vegan Diet: 21 Days of Vegan Recipe Menu Plans and 60+ Recipes (Vegan Diet to Lose Weight)

ISBN 978-1-989787-13-7

All rights reserved. No part of this guide may be reproduced in any form without permission in writing from the publisher except in the case of brief quotations embodied in critical articles or reviews.

Legal & Disclaimer

The information contained in this book is not designed to replace or take the place of any form of medicine or professional medical advice. The information in this book has been provided for educational and entertainment purposes only.

The information contained in this book has been compiled from sources deemed reliable, and it is accurate to the best of the Author's knowledge; however, the Author cannot guarantee its accuracy and validity and cannot be held liable for any errors or omissions. Changes are periodically made to this book. You must consult your doctor or get professional medical advice before using any of the suggested remedies, techniques, or information in this book.

TABLE OF CONTENT

Part 1 1

Introduction 2

Chapter 1 – What Is Vegan Eating? 4

Chapter 2 – Different Types Of Vegetarians 8

Chapter 3 – Health Benefits And Food Choices 15

Chapter 4 – Vegetarian Diet Myths 24

Chapter 6 – 5 Day Sample Diet 44

Chickpea Salad Wrap 46

Super Easy Veggie Chili 47

Sunflower Seed Oatmeal 48

Spinach Citrus Salad With Avocado 49

Grilled Veggie Pizza 50

Simple Peanut Butter And Banana Toast 51

Couscous Veggies And Bean Salad 51

Sweet Potato Asparagus Melts 52

Favorite Whole Grain Cereal And Almond Milk .. 53

Whole-Wheat Sesame Noodle Salad (Served Warm Or Cold) 53

Zucchini Lasagna 54

Toasted Avocado Bun 55

Spinach Quinoa Salad 56

Spaghetti Spinach Surprise 57

Ants On A Log 57

Conclusion 60

Part 2 64

Introduction 65

Chapter 1: Vegan Versus Vegetarian 69

ALL VEGANS ARE THE SAME, RIGHT? 71
ARE ALL VEGETARIANS THE SAME? 72
HOW DO VEGANS CONSIDER VEGETARIANS? 74
IS THIS PRESSURE NOT UNLIKE A VEGAN? 75
MAY A VEGAN EAT PRODUCTS LABELLED FOR VEGETARIANS? 78

Chapter 2 Why Become A Vegan? 80

1. A Lower Risk Of Type Two Diabetes And Heart Disease .. 82
2. Reverse Or Treat Other Health Conditions 82
3. Get Slim And Stay That Way Without Effort 84
4. Show Compassion And Kindness To Conscious Beings 85
5. World Hunger And Resources 86
6. Animal Products Can Be Dirty 87
7. We Do Not Need Animal Products 89
8. Save Our Environment And Halt Climate Change 90
9. An Amazing New Cuisine 91
10. Improved Fitness 92
11. Beautiful Skin And Better Digestion 93
12. Boost And Improve Your Mood 94
13. Save Money 95
14. It Is Easier Than Ever Before 96

Chapter 3 A Vegan Diet Outlined 97

WHAT CONSTITUTES THE VEGAN DIET? 97
WHAT CONSTITUTES A WELL-BALANCED, HEALTHY VEGAN DIET? ... 98
Nuts, Seeds And Legumes 98
JUST HOW HEALTHY CAN A VEGAN DIET BE? 101
Pay Attention To These Nutrients 102
How About Protein? 106
How About Calcium? 108

Chapter 4 How To Make The Transition To Veganism 110

GATHER ENOUGH INFORMATION 111
ADD TO YOUR EXISTING DIET BEFORE SUBTRACTING FROM IT 112
SEEK AND KEEP IN MIND YOUR STRONGEST MOTIVATION FOR THE CHANGE 113
KEEP UP YOUR POSITIVE ATTITUDE 114
START TO PLAN YOUR TRANSITION 115
From Vegetarian To Vegan 115
From Omnivore To Veganism, A Slow Transition 115
Gradually Reduce Intake Of Animal Product 115
Vegan All Out 116
GUIDELINES AND IDEAS FOR DIFFERENT APPROACHES 116
From Vegetarian To Vegan 117
From Omnivore To Veganism, A Slow Transition 117
Go Vegan All Out 118
FOOD BARRIERS AND THE IDEA OF ALL OR NOTHING 120
Focus On Barrier Foods Last 122
HELPFUL REMINDERS AND HINTS 124

Chapter 5 How To Budget For A Vegan Lifestyle 125

ALWAYS COMPARE PRICES 126
Frozen Versus Fresh 126
Bulk Versus Packaged 127

Organic Versus Non-Organic *128*
Brand Name Versus Generic Brand *128*
Compare Different Grocery Stores.................................... *129*
Consider Membership At A Good Wholesaler *130*
Search For Cheaper Options Of Super Foods And Vegan Specialty Foods Items *131*
Markdowns In Grocery Stores *131*
Online Retailers *132*
PREPARE AND COOK YOUR OWN FOOD 133
Prepare Your Convenience Meals At Home *133*
Concentrate On Whole Foods For Your Diet..................... *134*
MAKE THE MOST OF YOUR TRIP TO THE STORES 137
Staples Stock-Up.. *137*
Schedule Your Shopping Trips... *137*
BUILD YOUR OWN BUDGET LIST FOR GROCERIES 138

Chapter 6 Frequently Asked Questions............................ 140

1. Is It Difficult To Become A Vegan?................................. *140*
2. Is It Expensive To Be A Vegan? *142*
3. Are 99% Vegan Foods Acceptable? *142*
4. Which Are The Hidden Animal Ingredients?.................. *143*
5. What Is The Feeling About Silk And Honey?.................. *144*
6. How Do I Cope With Food Allergies?............................. *144*
7. I Felt Unhealthy On My Vegan Diet. What Went Wrong? *145*
8. Is It At All Possible To Eat Too Much?............................ *147*
8. Is It At All Possible To Eat Too Much?............................ *147*

Conclusion 149

About The Author.. 153

Part 1

Introduction

It doesn't matter if you are young or old, fit or out of shape, pregnant or going through menopause, the vegan diet done right will keep your body transform slim and strong. Whether you want to lose weight, fight disease, prevent animal cruelty, protect the environment, or just gain energy this guide is for you. In this introductory book you will discover everything you need to know about the Vegan Diet for Beginners to make your smooth transition into healthy living for life.

You'll learn about everything from the pros for strict vegan eating and the environmental benefits, to the ethics involved and how you can use this eating style to lose weight and improve your health. The disadvantages are also discussed along with solutions to any shortcomings you may come across. To verify the credentials of adopting a vegetarian lifestyle you will read from credible sources in the nutrition profession. The take-action information you learn will inspire you to make it happen. And the sample menu plan gives you the vision required to SEE it through.

There is no one PEFECT diet for everybody and you only know by trying. This book convincingly delivers so you can see that the massive vegan movement steadily gaining momentum world-wide, just may prove to be the best move for you.

Chapter 1 – What is Vegan Eating?

Vegan eating is documented to have begun before the 2nd millennium BC, according to animalliberationfront.com. Hindu beliefs state a diet void of meat and animal products is optimal for spiritual enlightenment. European vegans in ancient times were called "Pythagoreans," after the meat abstaining philosopher Pythagoras.

Numerous groups emerged vegetarian for both nutritional and ethical reasons. Monks are an example of a group that historically practice a vegan lifestyle, and it wasn't until 1846 the term "vegetarian" was coined. It comes from the Latin word "vegetus," which means "lively." And interestingly the English word "vegetable" meant a person that didn't eat flesh.

Europeans were the first to support and honorably promote the vegetarian diet. In the early 1900s The International Vegetarian Union was established. And more recently throughout the 20th century this lifestyle is growing because of strong ethical and moral reasoning, nutritional, economic, and environmental considerations. Understanding vegan eating is different from vegetarian. With vegan eating there are no animal products eaten whatsoever, and that includes animal by-products like dairy products, skins, and furs.

India vegetarians make up more than 70% of the worldly population of vegetarians, where almost 42% of the Indian populous follow vegetarian eating. In the U.S., studies show up to 5% of people are vegans. This number is growing.

There are different types of vegetarians. But vegetarianism is essentially practicing a diet that has foods that come entirely or mainly from plant sources. Vegans eat a diet consumes nothing to do with animals. The staples for a vegan diet are grains, nuts, seeds, legumes, fruits, and vegetables. There are some vegetarians that consume no animal products and others that may eat dairy, fish, or eggs, according to cancer.org.

For many, choosing to follow a vegan lifestyle gives piece of mind in the battle against animal cruelty and the slaughtering of innocent animals when there are other sources of food available. Many people turn to vegan eating to get healthy and lose weight. The problem many face is that a calorie is a calorie and just because you aren't eating meat doesn't mean you're slipping into your old bikini anytime soon. Bread, pasta, French fries, junk food, pastries, and other boxed foods are just as dangerous when it comes to obesity and preventable disease, like diabetes.

However, armed with the right information and a take action plan to turn healthy vegan, you can reach your weight loss goals for life. Important to note, one of the main concerns with plant-only eating is getting enough complete protein. In short complete protein is namely from animals sources and contains all 20 amino acids (building blocks) essential to disease prevention and great health. With vegan eating it's tougher to get this complete protein because you have to combine partial proteins with your plant eating. Just like putting a puzzle together. If you don't understand how to make certain you are eating the right combinations of protein-based foods to create complete proteins, you are depriving your body and mind of optimal fuel to function.

This guide will simplify the process and make certain you know exactly what you need to do if you choose to adopt a vegan lifestyle.

Chapter 2 – Different Types of Vegetarians

This is a Vegan Diet for Beginners book but it's very important you open your mind to all aspects of vegetarian eating. This will help you to better understand what vegan eating is and how it can benefit your mind, body, and life.

Over the years many different types of vegetarians have emerged. If you looked at a master list there's literally hundreds. We are going to zone into the four main types to start. These are recognized worldwide and provide the information you need to open your mind and get informed about vegetarian eating.

Livestrong.com states the four most recognized forms or vegetarianism are Semi-Vegetarian, Lacto-Ovo Vegetarian, Lacto-Vegetarian, and Vegan.

Semi-Vegetarian

Someone who chooses this style of vegan eating consumes meat on occasion, just not regularly. Often this type of plant-based eating is a stepping stone for people looking to eventually transform into true vegans, where no meat or animal products at all are eaten or used.

An advantage to Semi-Vegetarian eating is you won't have to worry about being protein deficient because your occasional meat meal will eliminate the worry.

Lacto-Ovo Vegetarian

This is the practice of vegetarian eating where no meat, fish, or poultry is allowed but other animal products like eggs (ovo), cheese (lacto), and milk are permitted. This type of vegetarian eating doesn't support the eating of animal flesh of any kind.

Lacto-Vegetarian

When you choose to become Lacto-Vegetarian you don't eat any sort of animal flesh or eggs, but you will eat other animal by-products, like milk, cream, butter, cheese, and yogurt. For most people choosing this style of plant eating is an ethical decision. They often believe animal life begins with the egg.

Vegan

If you want to fully commit to a vegetarian lifestyle you'll opt for Vegan eating. Medicalnewstoday.com states true Vegans won't eat any sort of food with animal origin, which includes honey, where a vegetarian may choose to consume eggs (lacto-ovo), or dairy (lacto). You can think of Vegan as the base or foundation of plant-based eating, the main event. Any other sort of classification of vegetarian eating are all parts of this main concept. Many of which are dependent on health goals and ethical beliefs.

Vegan goes a little further to stand strong against products made from animals, like leather, wool, makeup, creams, and any other consumer products that have animal testing to ensure they are safe for human use. Many of these controversies end up the main event on social media platforms, particularly when you see a celebrity sporting real fur.

REASONS MOST PEOPLE ADOPT THE VEGAN CONCEPT

Health and Wellness

There is good and bad in everything and many people believe eliminating meat from their diet will help them lose weight and get healthy. That's a logical theory but it's not how it works. What matters is what amount of food you are eating and what choices you are making. Are you eating fried burgers and breaded chicken? Or are you choosing poached salmon and barbecued chicken in moderation?

There are unhealthy ways to prepare and serve meat and animal products just the same are there are for plant choices. If you eat an unhealthy diet in general and choose to make healthy vegetarian choices, plenty of steamed veggies, legumes, and whole grain carbohydrates in moderation, you will lose weight.

But there are obese plant eaters because they choose to eat unhealthy in general and too much of it.

What I'm saying is you need to understand it's not meat that makes you unhealthy, it's what you are eating, how you are preparing it, and how much of it you are eating that does.

On that note, nutritionists report in the *Journal of Agricultural Food Chemistry* that many vegans are lacking vitamin B12. Some people have difficulty absorbing the plant-based version of this vitamin for a variety of reasons. Often taking a supplement reverses this issue.

Environment

Many environmentalists stand strong against the devastating effect animal farming has on our planet. Vegans don't believe the benefits outweigh the cost when considering the land the animal's need, the waste they pollute the environment with, the chemicals and pesticides used, and the water contamination that's inevitable when mass producing animals. The belief is that all of the resources being used to take care of these animals could be used for people instead. A personal choice.

Ethical and Moral Beliefs

Animal rights activists are the first to hop on the bandwagon condemning people that choose to eat meat and animal byproducts. The main belief is that killing animals is wrong and not essential for survival. People who are animal rights activists believe strongly in the rights of animals to live and not be slaughter for food.

The cruelty in which this animal processing is done converts many people to vegan eating. These animals are often pumped full of growth hormones and drugs to help them produce more, get bigger faster, and not get sick. For true vegans it's not just about the rights of animals, it's a lifestyle choice, a way of life that looks to alternative measures for food, void of any and all things "animal-related."

By understanding the different types of vegetarians abroad you open your mind to opportunity and finding what fits for you.

Some people just can't go all or nothing and that's perfectly fine. The idea is to figure out your reasons why you'd like to transform vegetarian first and then figure out what works for you.

This process isn't absolute and you need to remind yourself of this. Experts from the *ANA, American Nutrition Association* state people that set solid expectations when trying to create healthy eating habits are more likely to fail because reasonable expectations haven't been accepted.

This just means it's important to keep an open mind and set your goals, but also keep your mind open to make adjustments as you are working toward your goals. Two steps forward one step back is often how it works. When you expect this you increase your odds at succeeding. Just a little something to think about.

Up next are the health benefits in vegan eating.

Chapter 3 – Health Benefits and Food Choices

Weightlossresources.com reveals studies who that when vegans follow a balanced low-fat fiber-rich plant-based diet they naturally have lower risks for obesity, heart disease, high blood pressure, and various forms of cancer.

In general, vegan eating is lower in fat and calories because the wholesome foods associated are fruits and vegetables, versus higher fat meats, milk products, and breads and cereals.

Fat Associated with Animals...SATURATED

Fat Associated with Plants...UNSATURATED

Health Benefits

Losing weight, increasing energy, deterring disease, and lowering blood pressure and cholesterol are just a few of the reasons people get excited to turn to vegan. Let's look at the health benefits closer.

Heart - Too much saturated fat found in animal products is linked to high cholesterol, blood pressure, and ultimately heart disease, according to experts at womenshealthmag.com. Heart disease is the number one killer of women, which can be decreased significantly with a vegan lifestyle.

Studies show that even a small reduction in this bad fat intake will improve heart health.

Cancer - *The Canadian Cancer Society* states people that consume red and processed meats have the highest risk of developing cancer. Numerous research connects high-fat meats with liver, prostate, breast, and pancreatic cancer. Adopting vegan eating will help reduce the risk if you choose to go HEALTHY vegan.

Lose Weight - Meat has loads more calories and fat than plant food options. Which means it's more likely for you to be overweight if you are eating the higher fat food options, like meat and meat products. Nutritionists state numerous studies show people that eat meat as a staple in their diet are ten times more likely to be overweight than vegans. Add to that the fact that meat eaters also show a lifelong trend of gaining more weight as the years tick by.

In other words it's safe to say opting for health vegan eating will help you slim down for life.

Mental Plus - How you think and feel is extremely important in health and wellness. If your mind is cluttered and unhealthy because you are eating crap food, your outlook in life isn't going to be positive.

Psychology Today says a positive mindset isn't just about doing what makes you happy, it's also directly related with the food you eat and the lifestyle you live. When you eat a fatty burger and fries you may feel great a few minutes after because of all the simple sugar energy, but it won't take long for you to sink to the bottom of the barrel and feel like crap. Your sugars will drop and so will your energy, leaving you feeling lethargic and crappy.

Choosing a healthy low-fat diet will help boost your energy and flip your switch to positive. This is going to reflect positively in how you conduct yourself, your relationships at work and with your family and friends, the positive risk choices you take in life, and the smart healthy direction in which you lead your life.

Energy - This is one of the most immediate benefits of choosing to go healthy vegan. Fueling your body and mind with all-natural unprocessed PURE energy will send your energy levels straight through the roof. You will provide your internal systems with energy that lasts, leveling blood sugars and getting rid of those de-energizing mood swings most of us suffer at some point in the day. A constant source of quality energy will equate to feeling like a million bucks from the minute you wake up until after your head hits the pillow.

Basic Foods for Vegan Eating

*Vegetables and Fruits - You can pretty much eat as much as you what. Just remember variety is key and always look to try new combinations.

Serving Size - 1 cup of fresh fruit or vegetables, 1/4 cup dried

10-12 servings per day

Breads and Cereals - Whole wheat bread, rice, pasta, and crackers, along with steel cut oats. You need to be sure you are getting whole grain because this means there is little if any processing where the nutrients are stripped. Quick rolled oats are refined and not the best option, but they are better than opting white bread!

Serving Size - 1 slice bread, 3/4 cup cooked cereal, 3/4 cup rice or pasta, 5-6 crackers

6-8 servings per day

*Soy and Dairy-Free Products - This includes things like soy milk, almond milk, rice milk, and coconut milk. Add to that soy yogurt and dairy-free cream cheese, cheese (soy), margarine, and cottage cheese. There is also an organic vegan egg substitute called Emerg-G Egg Replacer. Look for organic products that are all natural. More and more vegan friendly foods seem to be introduced every day.

Stick with the proper serving size and choose low-fat when you can.

Serving Size - 1 vegan egg replacement, 2x2 inch cube soy cheese, 1 tbsp. margarine, 1 cup almond milk, 3/4 cup soy yogurt, 1/2 cup soy ice-cream

2-3 servings per day

Seeds, Nuts, and Legumes - Eating a nice variety is important. Peanuts, walnuts, almonds, cashews, sesame seeds, flax seed, kidney beans, chickpeas, sunflower seeds, lentils, peas, and soya beans are all healthy examples.

*Serving Size - 6-8 almonds, 1/4 cup sunflower seeds, 1/3 cup mixed nuts, 3/4 cup kidney beans, 3/4 cup peas

2-3 servings per day

With vegan eating the diet is low in saturated fat, high in fiber, and has plenty of healthy complex carbs from fresh fruits and veggies. Vegetarian eating is truly beneficial to great health if you choose to understand how to eat it right!

Beverages

When it comes to keeping your body hydrated the best source is water. Experts recommend 6-8 glasses of water each day to start. I think that's a little on the low end particularly if you are exercising daily, which of course I know you are!

All of your internal systems including brain function are dependent on adequate water stores. If you are dehydrated you'll feel tired and draggy, your skin may get dry and you're just going to feel crappy. With severe hydration your organs will shut down and eventually you'll slip into a coma and then death. So drink up!

Clear vegan-friendly soups and tea are also great options for making sure you've got lots of liquid energy in your body morning to night.

And when it comes to alcoholic beverages they don't really help you out. Alcohol dehydrate you, is often loaded will simple sugars and lots of calories. If you are going to have a drink on occasion stick to light beer or a mixed drink with a diet beverage, like rye and diet coke, or vodka and diet ginger-ale. Fancy mixed drinks are a nightmare!

Another no-no is fruit juices. They are loaded with sugar and calories, both of which are not going to help you lose weight and get healthy.

Note - If you are looking to lose weight it's very important you stick with the serving sizes. For most people it's about retraining your brain to expect less than those huge restaurant portions, often 3-4 times the amount your body really needs.

If you ate your meal and are still hungry don't be afraid to have an extra serving of veggies or a fresh piece of fruit. STARVATION is not healthy and it's won't get you to your weight loss goals.

Weightlossresources.co.uk nutrition experts report that when you sink into "starvation mode" your body intrinsically fights against starvation by becoming super-efficient at using as little energy as possible and saving as much as it can. This is meant to protect your fat stores instead of burn them, slowing your metabolism down considerably. Think of it like you would turning the heat down as much as you can to save money.

Most people want to do the opposite and rev up their metabolism to blast fat, which means the more your body can trust you will feed it regularly the better. Eat your healthy snacks and meals and your body WILL reward you.

Chapter 4 – Vegetarian Diet Myths

There's always someone out there to spoil the party! Vegetarian eating has its fair share of mistruths that we are going to debunk once and for all. Time to get to the facts on the vegetarian diet.

Myth 1 - There's no protein in plant sources

Straight up that's a heck of a lot of hogwash. Almost every natural food out there has a least a little bit of protein. Where the confusion arises is that in general animal sources have more protein than plant ones. On top of that most plant sources have incomplete proteins. So you have to eat them in combination to provide your body with all the protein it requires to stand strong.

Choosing every day to eat a wide variety of nuts and seeds, legumes, and soy milk products will give you all the protein you need to get healthy!

Myth 2 - Forget the gym if you're eating a vegetarian diet

If baseball all-star Hank Aarons and tennis sensation Venus Williams are vegetarian I don't think you have to worry about this eating style interfering with your gym routine. Truth is getting enough protein to build lean muscle when you're training is a little more difficult when you aren't eating meat, but it's definitely possible. It just takes a good understanding of what vegetarian eating is and making sure you are giving your body all the 20 amino acids it needs for complete protein to use for energy.

Myth debunked!

Myth 3 - Eating vegetarian guarantees you will lose weight

If you choose to eat plant sources only but also continue to consume high-fat processed foods you aren't going to lose weight. It's not just what you eat that's important but how you are preparing it and in what amounts. Whether you are only eating salads or beef, both can help you lose weight or gain it.

Myth 4 - Vegetarian eating will break the bank

If you are a smart shopper you can actually save money by removing meats. Yes fresh produce can get expensive, particularly when you are eating lots of it, but you can always opt to reduce your cost by shopping the reduced rack or opting for frozen.

Myth 5 - Vegetarian eating is all or nothing

Not true! Anything is better than nothing when you are choosing to improve your health and wellness. The new trend is where people are vegetarian but choose to have meat a few times a year. Remember we are trying to make an easy transition here. So for now there are no absolutes with vegetarian eating. Choose what works for you and open your mind to trying new tactics until you figure out what fits for you! Open your mind to letting go of meat. But don't beat yourself for having a piece of meat once in a blue moon otherwise you may feel deprived and snap back into the same old meat diet

Myth 6 - You're going to be weak and hungry eating vegetarian

Not sure where this one started but it certainly wasn't from a vegetarian that knew what they were doing. Vegetarian eating will provide ample vitamins, minerals, and energy if you do it right. Yes, if you are trying to lose weight by essentially starving yourself eating vegetarian, then you are going to be weak, tired, and always hungry. But if you create a sensible eating plan with plant-based foods and provide adequate calories for your body, then you've got nothing to worry about.

Myth 7 - Eating vegetarian is dull and boring

You seriously need your butt kicked if you believe that! With vegetarian eating you get to load your plate up with colorful and tasty fresh fruits and veggies. Tossing some nuts, sunflower seeds and lemon zest into your lentil salad is exciting! There are zillions of ways to make your vegan eating adventurous if you want to.

Making sure you are dealing with the facts is only going to help you make better choices for you. If something doesn't make sense to you with vegan eating make sure you find out the truth. Ask your healthcare provider, trainer, or do your own research to dig to the truth. Losing weight is tough enough when you've got the facts!

Chapter 5 – Tips to Vegan Eating and Superfoods

Change is tough no matter which way you slice it. Creating a new habit takes up to 6 months of repeating an action according to experts at *WebMD*. What you are looking to do is commit to trying something new like vegan eating. Then you've got to consciously make an effort to repeat these new actions daily until eventually they transform into habit and you don't have to think about them.

Here are a few pointers to help you make the change to vegan eating as smooth as possible.

Commit to the Idea

Unless you seriously want to become vegan you might as well stop before you waste your time. We both know making changes is hard and unless you commit to the change it will be short-lived or not happen at all. Do it for yourself and not for any other reason. If you are going vegan to try and impress a guy, to make your partner happy, or because all your friends are doing it you better think again.

Commit to see it through. Vegan eating may not be right for you but you've got to seriously try it to figure that out.

Open your mind

An open mind is a beautiful one. You might try something and fail and that's okay. But if you don't open your mind to try something new, like plant-based eating, you will never know what could have been. Choose to think positively because ultimately your belief becomes your reality. If you truly believe you are going to love vegan eating, chances are you will.

Set yourself up time-wise

If you are going to be cooking it's important to give yourself a little bit of extra time to craft your newfound way of eating. It's not routine yet so you will need to find yourself a few extra minutes to prepare your meals. The designing of your meals may take a little extra time because you've got to be a little more creative getting your complete proteins.

Buy the staples

Make sure you get to the market to fill your fridge and cupboards with everything you're going to need to eat vegan. The fresh produce you will need to shop for at least once a week but the rice, beans, cereal, and pasta you can store much longer.

Before you start just make sure you have everything you need to eat healthy vegan-style.

Stay away from fast food convenience

If you're going to pull the lazy card and buy a bunch of frozen meat-free pizza, burritos, and dinners you might as well hang your vegan hat up before you even start. Eating healthy whether vegan or not requires effort. Fresh is always better than frozen and creativity and different is the key to making your tummy and taste buds sing.

Don't try and hide the fact you are vegan when out

If you happen to head out with friends to eat don't be afraid to ask the wait staff for healthy vegan options. And I'm not talking cheese-less nachos or deep-fried bean burritos. You might as well join the crowd and have some fries and chicken wings.
Most restaurants will make just about whatever you like. Ask and you shall receive.

Be prepared before you head out the door

Make sure you've got plenty of meatless snacks prepped and ready to go BEFORE you head out the door. Slice and chop your veggies up for easy snacks, have plenty of fresh fruit around, and low-fat low-sugar all-natural granola bars. These make great snacks to throw into your bag when you're set to head out the door.

Understand this isn't all or nothing

Everyone screws up now and then, I don't care who you are. If you happen to head out with your friends and accidentally on purpose eat a piece of meat pizza, let it go! It's really not a big deal in the big picture. Think of it as a learning curve to help you make better decisions down the road. Besides, the "meat" on that pizza likely wasn't even REAL meat. Even worse I guess - lol.

Keep it to yourself

It's great that you are looking for a positive lifestyle change but that doesn't mean it will be something everyone else is going to agree with or even see positively. That's just life. So don't try pushing your views on other people, lecturing, or making people feel bad about their decisions just because they don't jive with yours. Stay positive but keep your thoughts to yourself with this one unless someone is seriously interested in learning about vegan eating.

One step at a time

I'm sure you are familiar with the average Joe that decides to start working out and just jumps off the couch one day and commits to slugging it out 2 hours a day at the gym.

TOO MUCH TOO SOON!

Chances are pretty good that although in theory this was a good thing, but the practicality of it just doesn't work. Easing yourself into things normally increases your odds at succeeding. There's nothing wrong with slowly phasing meat out of your diet one day at a time.

Set your goals and stick to them

You know you and it's important to set attainable goals for yourself. If you are transitioning yourself into full vegan eating you may want to give yourself a goal of 2 weeks to phase out your fast-food meat eating routine, and another two weeks to get rid of meat altogether. Whatever you do make it reasonable and positive for YOU!

Don't be an unhealthy vegan

It's just too easy to have the right intentions switching over to vegan eating, and just make bad food choices. I have friends that are classic examples. They initially switched to vegan eating to try and lose weight, only to fall prey to a junky meatless eating style. High-fat breads and cereals, chips, cookies and pastries were on the menu, and they look and feel crappy because of this.

Whether you choose to eat meat or not is your business. Just make the commitment to opt for healthy eating in the big picture and your body will thank you for it.

Commit to learning everything you can about vegan eating

The more you can cram into your brain about vegan eating the better. Information is knowledge and knowledge is power. By finding the time to research your chosen eating style you are only going to discover measures to help you improve upon the positive changes you have already made. Your health is important so make the time to update it regularly.

Junky eaters may need to eat A LOT more

If you traditionally eat even moderate amounts of unhealthy high calories fatty foods, the chances are pretty good you'll discover you've got to eat a heck of a lot of healthy vegan food to keep your tummy from rumbling.

This makes sense because typical plant-based vegan food is lower in calories and fat and this means the energy will scoot through your system faster than the fatty foods you are used to eating.

For example:

Hamburger (no cheese or condiments) and Small Fries - 500 calories - 20 grams of fat

2 cups Broccoli Ginger Avocado and Peanut Stir Fry - 250 calories - 5 grams of fat

The above example shows you just how much more food you get for less calories and fat. A nice surprise when you are committed to making a healthy habit out of eating vegan style.

Having a plan and the information you need to understand all aspects of the vegan diet is critical in long-term success. Use these pointers to help you open your mind and set yourself up for success. And I challenge you to continuously search for more.

Superfoods

Great News! There are some excellent superfoods in vegan eating that you need to know about. Simple easy foods that will help your body perform when you need it. Some of these you may be familiar with and I'm sure there's a few that will be new to you!

Avocado - It's true saturated animal fats often clog arteries, which may lead to stroke or heart disease. Research shows the fat in plant foods is critical to great health. Avocados help keep your skin and hair looking beautiful and also reduce the risk of cardiovascular disease. You will also get the added benefits of potassium, folate, and vitamin E and K.

Avocado is great in salads, stir-fry's, on sandwiches or crackers, or as a dip for just about anything!

1/4 of a large avocado is the recommended serving.

Walnuts

Walnuts are loaded with essential omega-3 fatty acids, zinc, iron, and protein to name a few. Experts recommend 2-3 servings of omegas each week to attain optimal health. Toss a few in your stir-fry, salad, yogurt, or just eat them in a dried fruit and nut mixture.

Quinoa

Quinoa is a hidden protein gem for vegetarians. It's the only plant source of complete protein and tastes great in anything from wraps and salads, to soups and even in potatoes. This is one complex carbohydrate grain you want on the menu.

Oatmeal

Peta.org says oatmeal can lower your cholesterol up to twenty percent! Oatmeal is a fabulous source of healthy carbohydrates and plant protein. Spice it up a notch or two by adding raisins, nuts, walnuts, or dried fruit. YUMMY!

Goji Berries

Ecorazzi.com says these berries, also known as the wolfberry, are a nutritional winner. They are loaded with antioxidants to help fight disease and some studies suggest they help fight off Alzheimer's. Add to that goji berries have 18 amino acids, 8 of which are essential, and more than twenty trace vitamins and minerals. They look like large raisins and you can eat them alone, in salads and stir-fry's, or even in a nut mixture.

Lentils

You won't have to worry about lacking fiber if you are eating plenty of lentils. They also provide your body with healthy folate, fiber, magnesium, and B vitamins. Lentils are versatile and can be used as a side dish, added to soups or stew, and even wraps or stir-fry's.

Berries

Load up on the protective antioxidants with berries. Blueberries, raspberries, strawberries, blackberries, and elderberries are bright and healthy to eat every day. Some of the nutrition in these berries are folate, magnesium, potassium, and vitamin K and A. Berries and yogurt or berries and oatmeal are fabulous ideas!

Sweet Potato

They are filled to the brim with minerals and vitamins, high in vitamin B6, C, D, iron, and potassium. Research shows sweet potatoes are excellent for verve function, bone, heart, and muscle health. Nutritionists report nearly 80% of the population is deficient in magnesium and sweet potatoes have oodles.

Tomato

Is it a fruit or a vegetable? Technically it's a fruit. Tomatoes are loaded with lycopene, powerful antioxidants that battle free radicals trying to fill your body with disease. Research shows by increasing lycopene you may reduce the risk of numerous cancers. Tomatoes are versatile and go with just about anything. You can have them in your salad or bake them in your lasagna. They taste great broiled and sprinkled with cheese, or just on their own.

Soy

The *National Cancer Institute* says soy is linked to reducing the risk of cancer and deterring heart disease. Tofu is a popular soy product. It's loaded with zinc and protein and often use as a meat replacement in recipes because of its texture. You can use tofu pretty much anywhere you'd use meat.

Pomegranate

I'm not going to lie, these are a pain in the butt to scoop. But they are well worth it because of all the ellagic acid and punic alagin they contain to fight off disease and support healthy skin. And I'll let you in on a little secret, if you look hard enough your grocer may have the seeds for sale and ready to eat!

Pomegranate seeds are bursting with flavor and can be enjoyed alone, in soy yogurt or with granola, in smoothies, or just in a fruit cup. Load them on and enjoy!

Kiwi

Kiwi is one of those fruits that often gets overlooked. It's a slightly sour fruit that has ample vitamin C, fiber, potassium, and vitamins A and E. *Shape* nutrition experts say that kiwi is one of the most nutritionally dense fruits. Eat them alone or add to your fruit cup, soy yogurt, or salad.

Chia and Flax Seeds

These seeds are rich in omega fatty acids, which help promote healthy brain activity and strong immunity. They also have protein, biotin, calcium, fiber, and potassium.

Grind them up and add them to your baking, sprinkle them in your oatmeal, or add them to your morning smoothie. YUM!

Knowing some of the best foods to eat when eating vegan will help you make the most of every bite. Contrary to what many people believe, the Vegan Diet is not all about carrot sticks and celery. There is such a wide range of satisfying tasty foods to choose from is overwhelming. Use this information as a base to explore and enjoy what vegetarian eating has to offer.

Time for us to apply!

Chapter 6 – 5 Day Sample Diet

This is an introductory book so we are going to use basic vegan eating as our sample diet. This means the only foods you aren't going to find are meats and animal products.

The first thing you need to do before you look at creating your diet plan is to figure out how many calories you need and what your goals are. For most people one of their goals with a lifestyle change is to lose weight, so we'll keep that in mind.

Calculating Calories

Online there are lots of different calorie counters you can use for free to figure out how many calories you need to sustain your weight. From there you can adjust your calorie intake if you want to lose weight, understanding there are approximately 3500 calories in a pound. Experts agree the most successful long-term weight loss incorporates healthier eating with regular exercise to increase the number of calories your body burns each day. Exercise will also naturally boost your metabolism to help you burn more energy even when you are resting.

In a nutshell these calorie counters take your age, height, weight, and sex, and then incorporate your activity level to come up with your BMI. Which is how many calories your body needs to stay at the same weight.

The *Dieticians of America* recommend approximately 2200 calories per day for the average female. So to keep our diet plan simple that's the figure we are going to use with our sample vegan diet plan.

Woman's Day nutritionists suggest eating 5-6 times per day to help keep your body energized, blood sugars level, and to encourage optimal calorie burn and craving control. Starving yourself between meals DOES NOT WORK!

On that note this plan will consist of 3 healthy meatless meals and 2 snacks per day to get you started. You may find for some reason this isn't enough food for you so you can adjust accordingly.

Breakfast Day 1

Energizing Sweet Green Smoothie

1 cup almond milk
2 cups fresh spinach
1 banana
1 cup fresh berries
1 scoop protein powder (optional)
Ice

Just toss all the ingredients in the blender for a super high-protein power breakfast loaded with essential vitamins and minerals your body needs. Adjust the thickness by adding more ice, or decreasing the milk amount.

Note - You can use 1/2 cup soy yogurt if you like to make it creamier.

Calories - Approx. 475

Lunch Day 1

Chickpea Salad Wrap

1 whole grain tortilla
1 cup mashed chickpeas with 1 tbsp. light mayo (dairy-free), spices, salt and paper to taste
Lettuce, tomato, cucumber, sprouts
1/4 cup dairy-free cheese

1 cup mixed raw veggies
Apple or pear
A whole grain chickpea salad wrap is simple and tasty. Just add any veggies you like to spice it up a few notches. Lots of fiber in the meal so make sure you're drinking lots of water!
Calories - Approx. 550

Dinner Day 1

Super Easy Veggie Chili

(just throw it all into the crockpot on med. for 2-3 hours)
1/4 cup diced onions
1/4 cup chopped carrots
1 clove minced garlic
1/4 cup green pepper
1/4 cup diced celery
1/2 tbsp. chili powder
1 can chopped tomato
1 can kidney beans with liquid
1 can chickpeas with liquid
1 cup corn
1 cup peas
Herbs to taste (cumin, parsley. basil)

1/2 cup non-dairy shredded cheese (sprinkle on just before serving
Serves 2
1 cup fresh fruit
This is a super easy dinner you can have ready when you walk in the door and it's awesome for leftovers. Stuff a tortilla with it with some non-dairy shredded cheese for lunch!
Calories - Approx. 600

Snack 1

Nut mixture (3/4 cup nuts, 1/4 cup raisins, 1/4 cup sunflower seeds)
Calories - Approx. 250

Snack 2

1 cup non-fat soy yogurt
1 cup fresh berries
Calories - Approx. 200

Breakfast Day 2

Sunflower Seed Oatmeal

1 cup steel cut oats
1 cup low-fat almond or rice milk

1/4 cup sunflower seeds
1/4 cup raisins
1 cup fresh fruit
The sunflower seeds add some zip to your oatmeal and the whole grains serve up long-term energy. Enjoy!
Calories - Approx. 450

Lunch Day 2

Spinach Citrus Salad with Avocado

2 cups fresh spinach
1 cup chunked oranges
1 cup sliced apple
1 cup diced cucumber
1/4 cup sliced almonds
1/4 cup sunflower seeds
1/4 cup diced avocado
1/2 cup raisins
2 tbsp. low-fat dressing
This is a simple but satisfying lunch. Lots of energizing iron from the greens, good fat from the avocado and almonds, and the raisins and sunflower seeds make it sweet and crunchy - YUM!
Calories - Approx. 600

Dinner Day 2

Grilled Veggie Pizza

1 large pita
1/2 cup chopped avocado
1 cup chopped spinach
1 sliced tomato
1/2 cup non-dairy cheese
1/4 cup chopped chives
1 tbsp. olive oil
1 cup canned tomato soup made with almond or coconut milk
Just brush the olive oil on and load the topping to grill on the barbecue or broil in the oven!
Calories - Approx. 550

Snack 1

2 cups air-popped popcorn
1 cup hot chocolate made with almond milk
Calories - Approx. 275

Snack 2

Peanut Butter Banana Smoothie - 1 ripe banana, 3/4 cup low-fat coconut milk, 2 tbsp. peanut butter, 1/4 cup soy yogurt
Calories - Approx. 350

Breakfast Day 3

Simple Peanut Butter and Banana Toast

2 slices whole grain bread
1/2 cup banana sliced
2 tbsp. all-natural peanut butter
A protein power packed breakfast to get you started off on the right foot. The banana adds a little extra flavor to the typical peanut butter and toast.
Calories - Approx. 400

Lunch Day 3

Couscous Veggies and Bean Salad

1 cup couscous prepared with organic veggie soup mix for flavor
1 cup broccoli steamed and chopped
1/2 chopped carrots
1/2 chickpeas
1/2 red kidney beans
1/2 cup corn

1 slice whole grain bread with 1 tbsp. nut butter
Calories - Approx. 500

Dinner Day 3

Sweet Potato Asparagus Melts

1 large sweet potato (baked, sliced in half lengthwise)
1/2 cup asparagus sliced
1/2 cup red pepper thinly sliced
1/2 cup mushrooms thinly sliced
1 cup shredded non-dairy cheese
2 cups garden salad with 2 tbsp. low-fat dressing
Spread veggies on sweet potatoes and sprinkle with non-dairy cheese and broil on low till golden (6-8 minutes).
Calories - Approx. 600

Snack 1

1 cup pretzels
Apple
Calories - Approx. 200

Snack 2

6-8 whole grain crackers
2 tbsp. non-fat dairy-free cream cheese
Small handful almonds
Calories - Approx. 250

Breakfast Day 4

Favorite Whole Grain Cereal and Almond Milk

1 cup of your favorite whole grain cereal
1 cup of almond or rice milk
1 cup fresh fruit of your choice
Talk about an easy tasty breakfast to get you energized for the day. Don't be afraid to double up on the berries to increase those antioxidants that protect you from disease! Yummy!
Calories - Approx. 500 calories

Lunch Day 4

Whole-wheat Sesame Noodle Salad

(served warm or cold)

3/4 cup cooked whole-wheat spaghetti
1 tsp sesame oil
1 tsp lime juice

1 tbsp. soy sauce
1 cup steamed snow peas
1 cup steamed beans
1/4 cup sliced green pepper
1/4 cup toasted sunflower seeds
1/4 cup toasted sesame seeds
1 cup of low-fat soy yogurt with 1/2 cup blueberries

Good warm or cold this nutritious wholewheat pasta salad is loaded with essential vitamins and minerals to fill you up for the long run.

Calories - Approx. 650

Dinner Day 4

Zucchini Lasagna

1 package fresh ready to bake lasagna noodles
1 cup tomato sauce
1 cup non-dairy cottage cheese (or cooked beans)
1 1/2 cup sliced mushrooms
2 cups sliced zucchini
2 cups shredded non-dairy cheese
8x8x2 inch pan

1 small sub bun sliced in half lengthwise and brushed with margarine or non-dairy butter substitute (broil till golden)

For the lasagna just preheat oven to 400 degrees Celsius. Layer noodles on bottom of pan, brush with sauce, spread 1/2 cup non-dairy cottage cheese, half the mushrooms and zucchini, 1 cup soy cheese, repeat and bake 30 minutes or until soy cheese is golden. Serves 4.

Calories - Approx. 650

Snack 1

1/2 whole grain bagel toasted with 2 tbsp. hummus
1/2 cup raisins
Calories - Approx. 200

Snack 2

1 cup carrots, celery, and cucumber
1/4 cup non-dairy creamy dressing
Calories - Approx. 300

Breakfast Day 5

Toasted Avocado Bun

2 small whole grain buns
1/2 avocado sliced or mashed
Banana

For the avocado bun it's best to toast the bun first and then spread with the avocado. This gives you a nice dose of healthy fat to start the day. And how can you go wrong with a tasty banana to top of your morning meal?

Calories - Approx. 350

Lunch Day 5

Spinach Quinoa Salad

2 cups spinach
1 cup quinoa
1/4 cup soy cheese
1/4 cup chopped pepper
1/4 cup chopped cucumber
1/4 cup cherry tomatoes
1/4 cup thinly sliced onion
1/4 cup sliced water chestnuts
2 tbsp. favorite low-fat dressing

Quick and tasty is what this spinach salad is all about. Did you know that quinoa is one of the only complete proteins that is

plant based? That makes this lunch perfectly balanced.
Calories - Approx. 550

Dinner Day 5

Spaghetti Spinach Surprise

3 cups spaghetti cooked, trained
1 cup tomato sauce
1 cup spinach
1/2 cup each cooked and sliced sliced carrots, celery, pepper, eggplant, broccoli
Serves 2
1 cup unsweetened apple sauce
This is a tasty dinner that's loaded with energizing carbs with staying powder. Warm the applesauce for some extra sweetness.
Calories - Approx. 700 calories

Snack 1

All-natural whole grain granola bar
Calories - Approx. 250

Snack 2

Ants on a Log

1 celery stalks
2 tbsp. all-natural peanut butter
1/4 cup raisins
Calories - Approx. 250

Note - It's important to always have a little something in your tummy to keep your energy levels up. This is a trial and error process and if you are seriously hungry just add an extra snack to your day. It won't take your system long to get used to your new vegan eating style so you can tune into your daily energy needs a little more accurately.

For instance, if you increase your exercise routine you will need to add at least another snack to provide the essential protein, good carb, and good fat energy to perform!

This menu plan should give you a solid base to get started. Don't be afraid to make adjustments to set yourself up for success. Only you know your body and how it processes food. If a particular food doesn't work then try another. Through trial and error you will better understand your system and how to provide to get the results you want.

Time for you to trust yourself and GO FOR IT!

Conclusion

The Vegetarian Times says more than seven million people world-wide follow vegetarian eating, and the number of vegans is increasing dramatically. In order to be successful you need to open your mind to change and WANT to make it happen.

This book provides you with the information you need to understand and take-action with the Vegan Diet for Beginners. Keep in mind if full vegan doesn't work for you there's always the option of vegetarian eating, which is a little more lax. Some forms of vegetarian eating allow people to eat products of animals like eggs, yogurt, cheese, and milk, which isn't permitted with strict vegan eating. Comfort foods which some people just can't seem to live without.

If you want to lose weight then my advice is to pay close attention to your daily caloric intake and make sure you get an hour of moderate to intense exercise 4-5 times each week. This could include 30-45 minutes of biking, running, swimming, or even fast walking. It's also important that you get at least 2-3 days each week of strength training/weight lifting exercises. This will help build your lean muscle mass which blasts fat and boosts you metabolism to burn more calories. And that's just a start.

By using the Vegan Diet to step-by-step make healthier food choices, combined with increased rigorous ROUTINE physical activity, your body will have no choice but to start shrinking and your energy levels will shoot straight through the roof.

Time for you to take action!

*COMMIT to changing your eating style for the better. Ditch the processed fast food crap for healthy wholesome plant-based vegan food.

*CREATE YOUR PLAN to get you there smoothly. If you need help this make sure you talk to a professional. Your doctor, nutritionist, or even fitness training will help you out.

*KNOW YOUR GOALS and mark them down so you consciously acknowledge them. If you don't have goals it's pretty tough to stay motivated to reach them.

*MEASURE your progress. Step on the scale, be wary of your clothing size, or just use your mood and energy levels to SHOW yourself eating vegetarian is a step in the right direction for you. If you can't SEE the progress you'll eventually fall of track.

*ACCOUNTABILITY is very important in the big picture. Let your friends and family know what you are doing, along with your doctor and anybody else that will hold you to this fabulous lifestyle change. It's easy to let yourself down but know so easy when you've other people to answer to!

*CHECK-IN with yourself regularly. It's important to realize sooner rather than later if you are steering off course. This may be something as simple as taking a look at your progress on a set day every week. If you do this you will be able to change your direction without wasting too much time.

*JOURNALS are excellent in making sure you are getting results for your actions. It may seem a little bit tedious but recording

EVERYTHING you eat at least for the first month is an excellent idea. This way you can see with your own eyes what works and what doesn't. And if you end up hitting a plateau or get stumped you can always scoot back through your notes and find where you made an error. It's just too easy to quit if you don't have some sort of record of what you are doing when trying to establish a new healthier way of eating.

*FOCUS ON THE POSITIVE and the negatives won't be such a big deal. As humans we are programed to look for things that are wrong naturally. By changing this and rewarding yourself by acknowledging what you are doing that is right, you will fuel your internal desire to want more. It's a choice and it works if you REALLY want it.

Looks like you've got a lot of work to do. Time for you to get started and know that you WILL succeed, just don't quit!

Good Luck!

Part 2

Introduction

Veganism is nothing new, although it really only has gained popularity in the last ten years or so. The term vegan was first used by Donald Watson who was the co-founder of the Vegan Society in 1944 in England. His idea of a vegan diet was different from what it is today; what he really meant by the term was someone who followed a non-dairy vegetarian diet. However, in 1951 he also proclaimed that he strongly rejects the use of animals as a

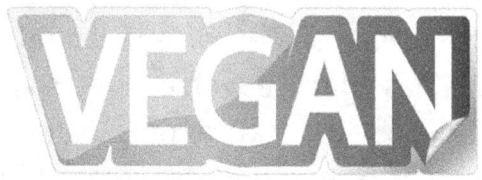

commodity and wants people to live their lives without exploiting animals.

Today vegans come in many different forms and categories. Although vegans generally abstain from consuming the flesh of animals, others also cut out all dairy and eggs from their diets. Some will eat fish and seafood while others only consume raw vegetables and fruit. But for many people around the world, veganism is much more than a healthy plant based diet. Most vegans avoid the use of any products which derive from animals, like leather shoes, bags, clothing etc. They do not approve of the industrial farming and slaughtering of animals. Some even avoid products that come from insects like silk and honey.

Leading a vegan lifestyle has numerous benefits. Maybe the most profound is our health. Eating a diet of animal fats and protein has many adverse effects on our body and is the cause of a number of illnesses like heart disease, hypertension, cancer, rheumatoid arthritis amongst others. By following a whole plant based diet, many of these conditions can be avoided. Vegetables, fruit, legumes and whole grains which all form part of the vegan diet contain no cholesterol at all and very little saturated fats. It is high in fiber and nutrition and many contain a high level of protein.

Veganism imposes less stress on our natural environment and improves our chances of saving the earth for future generations. The breeding and feeding of livestock to feed the masses is really a tremendously inefficient way of using our resources. Around sixty percent of deforestation has taken place to make room for agriculture. If everyone switches to a vegan diet, the products of this agricultural development can be used to feed people instead of livestock which we kill again for food.

Inhumane animal practices will more likely come to an end. People all over the world are becoming aware of the rights of animals and how they should be treated. The cruelty involved in the raising and slaughtering of many farm animals is not a secret anymore and many more people are opposed to these practices. The moral way to solve this problem is to switch to a plant based diet which is actually a lot healthier too.

In these modern times we live in, we definitely do not need animal products for our clothing, shelter or sustenance like our ancestors did. Therefore, there can be no good reason for not adopting a vegan lifestyle. It will only be to our benefit and future generations will thank us for our contribution in saving the planet.

~ Richard C.~

Chapter 1: Vegan versus Vegetarian

People often wonder what exactly constitutes the differences between vegetarianism and veganism and sometimes the two are even confused with each another.

In general vegans are considered to be similar to vegetarians, although in a different form, which is near the truth. However, vegans have a different viewpoint; they make a clear distinction between these two. The main reason for this is because various sub categories have developed under the overall umbrella of vegetarianism, some which include the consumption of meat and some animal by-products and vegans do not want to associate themselves with the latter.

Although the defining lines are quite clear, chefs, foodies and companies trading in food products often confuse them. Both vegans and vegetarians refrain from eating animal flesh. That includes chickens, cows, pigs or sea creatures. Other than vegetarians, vegans also do not eat dairy products, eggs, or any products deriving from animals, whereas vegetarians in general do not have an issue with consuming products like eggs, cheese, milk etc.

Vegans also feel strongly about the testing of products on animals and will not use them. These include skin creams, make-up and anything made from the skins of animals like leather shoes, bags and belts. As far as these kinds of products are concerned, vegetarians are more lenient.

The definition of a vegetarian is not that clear cut. Some vegetarians will eat eggs, but no dairy or you may encounter someone who would have no objection to wearing leather shoes, but would not eat any dairy products or eggs. On the other hand; a vegan is quite clear about his or her beliefs. They do not tolerate the consumption of animal flesh, the wearing of anything made from the skins of animals, or the use of products that were tested on animals. Vegans therefore believe in leaving animals alone; letting them get on with their lives without interfering or exploiting them.

All vegans are the same, right?

No, there are variations on the vegan diet, although the main ideas are the same. One branch of veganism, called the raw vegans will not touch food that has been cooked at temperatures more than forty-eight degrees Fahrenheit. This implies that most of their menu consists of raw foods like nuts, fruit and raw vegetables.

Another sub category calls themselves the Paleo vegans. Although they may eat meat and fish, they will abstain from dairy, all grains or processed foods. They base their diet on the foods which our ancestors from the Paleolithic era presumably ate. They also rely heavily on fruits and vegetables.

The majority (ninety-nine percent) of vegans try to eat organic, high quality food and avoid refined sugar products like sodas and sweets. This means that any ready-made meals or processed foods will be a no-go. Paleo vegans are considered by most as an extremely healthy kind of vegan.

Are all vegetarians the same?

Although vegetarianism started off as a clearly defined choice of dietary requirements, over the years this tree has sprouted many branches. The result of this was that vegans felt the need to dissociate themselves from this broad term of vegetarianism and form their own distinct, exclusive category.

I have to point out that the general term of vegetarianism does not always imply consideration for the welfare of animals since some groups even include meat in their diet and most allow animal protein in some form or the other. Vegetarianism can more aptly be described as a diet with the emphasis on the individual's health, whether it may be true or a presumption. This kind of diet will include or exclude foods on their apparent health value and not necessarily on the impact it has on the welfare of animals.

The typical vegetarian will often get annoyed with all these variations and distance himself from them.

Here are some of the major branches of vegetarianism:
- **Ovo-lacto** vegetarians will readily consume eggs and dairy products, but will abstain from fish and meat. This is considered the basic diet for vegetarians.
- **Lacto** vegetarians exclude fish as well as dairy products but also keep away from meat. They will eat eggs and are often called the eggetarians.
- **Ovo** vegetarianism means the exclusion of meat but allows for fish, vegetarian cheese as well as other products based on milk.

- **Flexitarians** (also called the semi vegetarians) refers to anyone who tries to reduce his consumption of meat. However, they will consume meat on occasions when they have the craving for it. This type of vegetarianism is mostly ridiculed and not considered in high regard.
- **Pollo** vegetarians exclude the flesh of animals and fish but will allow poultry, eggs and dairy. They are also called pollotarians.
- **Pesco** vegetarians follow a diet which include seafood and fish, dairy and eggs and on occasion poultry, but do not include the flesh of land animals. They are sometimes referred to as pescatarians.

How do vegans consider vegetarians?

Vegans in general do not have issues with their vegetarian brothers or sisters. At times, they might exhibit a slight frustration or disappointment with their peers' apparent lack of drive to follow through and become full-blown vegans.

In the eyes of vegans, vegetarians are teenagers on their way to becoming worthy adults; they consider veganism the next and ultimate step to full maturity. They will commend people who decided to become vegetarians but will stand in the wings, eagerly awaiting their transition to veganism. They sometimes find it difficult to see vegetarianism as the ultimate goal. So now you understand why your vegan friend has been nudging you all this time since you changed your diet to a vegetarian one; she is waiting for you to take the last and most important step!

Is this pressure not unlike a vegan?

One of the biggest differences between vegetarians and vegans is their regard for and attitude towards of animals. Where the majority of vegetarians do not really concern themselves with this issue, vegans really take it to heart. This is why some vegetarians will eat dairy products and make use of products made from animal skins. In a vegan's eyes, dairy industries are maybe the cruelest amongst the meat industries. They believe that cows are continuously tortured when their milk is being extracted and cannot tolerate it that the young calves are physically removed from their mothers right after birth.

It does not stop here: The male calves will be used as bulls for breeding purposes or slaughtered for veal whereas the females in time will become milk producers. Those that do not produce enough milk will be sold for meat. Have you ever had the unfortunate experience of hearing calves' calls when separated from their mothers or when they realize they are destined to be slaughtered? If so you will sympathize with vegans who will not touch dairy and are not very happy with other people doing it.

The poultry industry is another matter of great concern for vegans. Male chicks are considered superfluous and are killed in industrial blenders, electrocuted or gassed. Laying hens are never free to roam around in their natural environment but are cramped into tiny spaces where all they do is lay eggs. When their egg-laying days are over they are killed; their spines are snapped or their necks wrung.

This is another reason for vegans' intolerance of people who follow a vegetarian diet but do not progress to veganism. From this it is obvious that in the eyes of a vegan, animal rights are equally important to eating a healthy diet, if not more so.

Scientists agree that a well-balanced diet of veganism is the number one diet you can follow for good health. Still, vegans would gladly make sacrifices regarding their own health if it ensures that animals are allowed to live a peaceful, natural life; the kind Mother Nature would allow them to live.

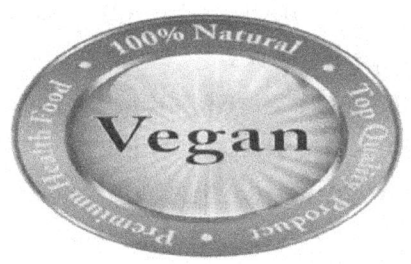

May a vegan eat products labelled for vegetarians?

No, 'vegetarian safe' does not mean 'vegan safe'. The guidelines provided by the FSA officially read as follow:

- Vegetarian: This term does not apply to foods which are from animals. Neither does it apply to any foods that were produced from or made with the help of any products that derive from animals, whether these animals have died, or were slaughtered, or have died as a consequence of being consumed.
- Animals: This term includes domestic, wild or farmed animals for instance livestock, game, poultry, shellfish and fish, crustaceans, tunicates, amphibians, molluscs, insects and echinoderms.
- Vegan: This term does not apply to any foods of animal origin. Neither does it apply to foods which have been produced from or made with the help of any animals or their products. This includes products coming from animals that are still alive.

You will agree that these guidelines are quite clear and straight forward. However, in the food industry these terms are more often than not used in a misleading manner. Often a product will be labelled as suitable for either vegans or vegetarians but in actual fact they are just the company's interpretation of that which they think is suitable.

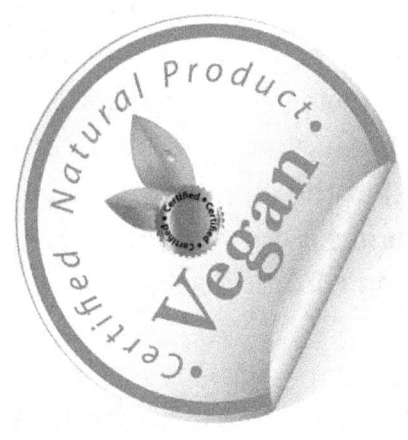

Chapter 2 Why Become a Vegan?

During the last few years veganism has grown in popularity all over the world. People of all age groups, professions and backgrounds have made the decision to drastically change their diet. It is apparent that a great number of people have realized that the longevity and compassion which comes with veganism is a better option than chronic diseases.

Only two years ago, it was reported by USA Today that almost fifty percent of the American people are attempting to eat less meat. On top of that, as many as a twenty percent of all students have become either vegans or vegetarians or are endeavoring to consume less meat. It surely seems as if it is becoming a trend, and there must be a good reason for it. So, why consider becoming a vegan?

Our diets impact greatly on our lives in many ways. It shows how aware we are of the world around us, whether we will suffer from certain diseases later in life and which companies profit from us. To put it simply, our power as consumers is greater than we realize; we can use or withhold our money to determine the success or downfall of large industries. However, the financial element is not the only one to consider.

I am sure you have already heard some of the arguments about the pros of veganism or a diet based on plants. Different people will need different reasons to motivate them towards a change in diet.

You may already be on the way to becoming a vegan or just thinking about it. Here are a few reasons which may help you decide.

1. A lower risk of Type Two diabetes and heart disease

In our Western world, these are probably the chronic diseases most commonly found. They are mostly man-made so in reality no-one should have to suffer them. It is really scary to think that the accumulation of plaque in the arteries begins unbelievably early on in life; around the age of ten.

The majority of health organizations agree that the cholesterol and saturated fats found in animal products are the main culprits that contribute to both diabetes and heart diseases. A diet which improves the condition of our arteries will do the same for diabetes Type 2. It may even play a role in reversing this type of diabetes.

2. Reverse or treat other health conditions

Nothing is more important than your health; good health surely is our greatest asset. Therefore, we should seriously consider any changes we can make to our life style in order to decrease and minimize our risk of diseases. We should assist our bodies in its endeavors to heal and improve our health. A great number of the health conditions we face are really within our control.

An increasing number of health organizations now condones a well-balanced vegan diet and during all the different stages of your life. They found that vegans show lower instances of increased blood pressure, cancer, high cholesterol, diabetes, cardiovascular diseases, and Alzheimer's.

Often this diet based on plant foods is more efficient than surgery and medication as far as these above-mentioned diseases are concerned. According to the World Health Organization, processed meat can cause cancer and is considered a carcinogen. Red meat, more than likely, is too and a China Study showed a clear connection between milk protein or casein and cancer. You can draw your own conclusion from this.

3. Get slim and stay that way without effort

The only people to average a healthy and normal body mass index are vegans. This is to be expected since an increase in the consumption of animal products equals an increase in BMI. Various reasons for this can be quite easily accounted for. Animal products are high in fat and very low in carbohydrates. These fats contain more calories; they are also easier transformed into body fats than those from carbs.

We can fill our dinner plates with vegetables and potatoes and still stay slim whereas the calorie density present in most animal products often leads to our overeating on calories. Animal products also naturally contain hormones to stimulate growth which is not beneficial to us. So, without having to starve yourself you can stay slim on a diet consisting of plants.

4. Show compassion and kindness to conscious beings

Some people do not consider the ethical arguments of veganism that important but still, kindness towards sentient beings cannot be ignored. Sparing the lives of others, especially innocent creatures, will always be the correct and moral thing to do. Unfortunately, through the years the dairy and meat industry have launched huge campaigns to brainwash consumers; to smooth their conscience. On food cartons, we see happy animals frolicking in the fields while that has nothing to do with the reality which is far more sinister. You must agree that there cannot be anything humane about farming with animals or slaughtering them.

The egg and dairy industries are equally guilty in this regard and work hand in hand with their meat counterparts. Dairy cows, after being forcefully impregnated, deliver calves which are taken away from them immediately after birth. The calves are slaughtered and the cows' milk extracted by machines. Eventually they end up in stores in the form of hamburger meat. And nobody can be immune to the sight of tiny male chicks discarded on garbage heaps, gassed alive or shredded like mere inanimate objects of no value.

5. World hunger and resources

Veganism does not only concern animals, it also has a huge impact on the lives of humans. Many people around the world suffer as a result of the demand for all kinds of animal products. You may ask how this is applicable. I will explain. The world population at present stands around seven billion. If it were not for all the grain (fifty percent of the total production) needed to feed animals in the meat industry, we would grow enough to feed up to ten billion people; more than enough so that nobody has to starve. At the same time, eighty-two percent of the children who live in the vicinity of livestock, are actually starving. This third world produced meat is then shipped off to the developed countries for consumption.

Livestock is fed about seventy percent of all the grain produced in the US, enough to feed eight hundred million human beings. Another factor is water. During the production of animal products, a massive amount of water is needed. Each vegan can save around 725,000 gallons of this precious liquid a year. Imagine then the impact these savings can have on our world.

6.Animal products can be dirty

Each time you bite down on a piece of meat, or dine on dairy products and eggs, you are ingesting known antibiotics, bacteria, dioxins, hormones and other toxins, all of which could lead to serious health risks in humans. Dangerous bacteria which live and breed in the intestines, feces and flesh of animals are found in high percentages of slaughtered flesh in this country. These contaminations include E. coli, listeria and campylobacter.

Seventy-five million instances of food poisoning are recorded every year, of which five thousand are fatal. According to USDA, seventy percent of these cases are a direct result of the contamination of animal flesh. A long history of pharmaceutical abuse on factory farms lead to the development of super bacteria strains which have become resistant to antibiotics. And it does not end here; there is another serious danger lurking in the flesh of farm animals. Roxarsone, the antibiotic most commonly used for dosing these animals contains serious amounts of a most toxic form of arsenic.

Another factor to consider is the development of cancer which can be caused by the hormones found in the flesh of animals. Obesity and enlarged breasts in males, or gynecomastia are also caused by the intake of animal hormones. Do not be misled by the 'organic' label on meat, it does not change much.

7. We do not need animal products

It is totally unnecessary to slaughter farm animals, and thus it becomes an act of cruelty. No proof exists that it is necessary for human beings to eat diary, eggs or meat to maintain good health and growth. Actually, the exact opposite is true. Over the years we have acquired this behavior and were taught which of the animals it is acceptable for us to eat. This is the complete opposite of wild animals like bears or lions that hunt instinctively and show different behavior when it comes to their choice of prey. As far as milk is concerned, we certainly need nothing more than our mothers' during our first years after birth.

No animal wants to die, they appreciate and love life but unfortunately, we see them only as a herd of faceless farm animals with no unique emotions or personalities unlike dogs and cats. Once we come to this understanding, that every animal is an individual and should be respected as such, can we understand the moral behind veganism and start aligning our actions with these ethical views.

8. Save our environment and halt climate change

Between eighteen and fifty percent of the pollution created by man derives from the meat industries. Factory farming contributes even more than transportation towards the greenhouse conditions we are facing today. Additionally, about forty calories of energy generated by fossil fuels are needed to manufacture one single calorie of beef. Only about two calories of this fuel are used to manufacture plant proteins.

Seventy-five kg of CO_2 emissions equal only one-pound hamburger meat; that is the exact same as driving your vehicle for three weeks.

Wild animals also suffer from the consequences of our meat eating habits; currently mass extinction threatens eighty six percent of mammals and birds and eighty eight percent of amphibians. We are losing many species as complete extinction stares them in the face in the not so distant future.

9.An amazing new cuisine

Think delicious quinoa salads, hearty bean burgers or a thick lentil soup to name only a few. Across the world, twenty-thousand species of plants, all edible, are just waiting for us to explore. Of these around two hundred have been farmed or domesticated. How many of these have you actually tried? Why not broaden your horizons and tantalize your own and your family's taste buds with new and exciting recipes? A whole new world is awaiting you. So, start experimenting.

Do not think that you will have to compromise on taste. Just find the correct replacements, for example bananas or applesauce for eggs, or use recipes that do not include animal products.

10. Improved fitness

Many people assume that they will lose muscle mass and energy if they refrain from eating animal products. This is far from the truth. Because dairy and meat are so difficult to digest, your body uses a lot of energy for the process, leaving you feeling tired. A plant based diet will not prevent you from achieving the levels of fitness you want to reach. On the contrary; it might boost your energy levels and your strength. Veganism can provide you with lots of protein and the very best nutrients.

It is not necessary to keep a close watch on your intake of protein, either; whole plant foods all contain protein of a high quality. You need around forty to fifty g per day and that can easily be gotten from green veggies, legumes, whole grains, seeds and nuts. Corn is eleven percent protein, rice eight percent, beans twenty seven percent and oatmeal fifteen percent.

A vegan diet with its low-fat content will help you to build muscles that are lean but strong, so no more 'bulking and cutting'.

11. Beautiful skin and better digestion

What very few people know is that these two things are closely connected. Dairy is often the worst culprit when it comes to acne. Physicians, who are on the whole oblivious of this, send you home with harsh chemicals and prescriptions for medication instead of looking at your diet. Our skin reflects our diet. If you cut down or eliminate all fatty foods like oils, animal products and even some kinds of nuts, you will soon see an improvement in the health of your skin.

Vegetables and fruits rich in water will provide your skin with that additional boost; they harbor high levels of minerals and vitamins. The fiber will assist with better digestion, as well as the elimination of some toxins, all resulting in a healthier skin.

12. Boost and improve your mood

Animals being lead to the slaughter produce an abundance of stress hormones and continue to do so right up to the end. Cutting out meat means that you rid yourself of these unnecessary hormones. It will have an immense effect on your own stability and mood. And that is not all.

For a long time now, we are aware that people on a diet of plants are in general in a better state of mind. They experience less anxiety, tension, anger, depression, fatigue and hostility. The high levels of antioxidants found in a vegan diet, especially veggies and fruit, is the reason for this improved state of mind. When this diet is combined with a low intake of protein and fat, it has additional benefits for someone's psychological wellbeing.

Foods rich in carbohydrates like oats, rye bread and brown rice help to regulate the levels of serotonin in our brains. As you well know, serotonin is an important controller of our moods. In the expanding and revolving scene of neurological studies, a diet based on plant foods might assist in the treatment of symptoms of depression and anxiety.

13. Save money

Meat is by far the most expensive component of the general diet whereas a vegan diet is extremely economical. If you concentrate on beans, grains, nuts, legumes, seeds and those veggies and fruits that are in season, you can cut your monthly budget for foodstuffs in half. Remember also that a lot of these are available in bulk. Most of them can be stored for long periods of time.

Think how much you can save with this diet instead of running into the deli for a double cheeseburger of sandwich packed with unhealthy ingredients. The options for a vegan diet are many fold and will fit any budget. Sticking to a healthy diet like this will decrease the risk of chronic diseases and may even prevent them.

Therefore, you will save a lot on medications and visits to your doctor.

14. It is easier than ever before

Since veganism has become popular amongst many people, it is more readily available. Maybe you just never noticed it before, but most supermarkets offer lots of vegan foods, like dark chocolate, Oreos, Twizzlers and Taco dinners. There are a wide variety of sauces, mixes and plant based options for milk, ice cream made from coconut milk and mock meat to name but a few. These changes of their customers' culinary preferences are reflected in the data; the sales of non-dairy products have gone through the roof, whereas the sales of meat alternatives will reach five billion dollars by 2020.

Restaurants have also caught on and many offer vegan dishes on their menus. Visit an ethnic restaurant, diner or food chain and you will be astonished at the variety of delicious dishes on offer these days.

Chapter 3 A Vegan Diet Outlined

What Constitutes the Vegan Diet?

This diet consists of food derived only from plants. A vegan does not consume or use anything which comes from animals. This includes eggs, milk and the flesh of animals. Vegans prepare and eat their food in the same kind of dishes as non-vegans, for instance soups, stir-fries, stews, casseroles and salads. Their diet includes a huge variety of food including the traditional favorites found in vegan versions like pizzas, burritos, tacos, burgers, barbeques and lasagna.

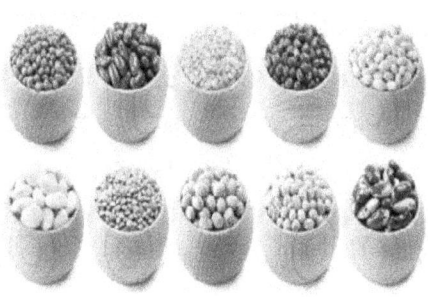

What Constitutes a Well-Balanced, Healthy Vegan Diet?

The 4 food groups that make up a healthy vegan diet are:
- Nuts, seeds and legumes
- Grains
- Fruits
- Vegetables

Your age, health condition and your activity level determine your energy requirements and nutrient needs. Every person's needs will differ; therefore, the following guide should be seen only as an example for a balanced diet.

Nuts, seeds and legumes
- Four or more servings daily

This group includes soy products, split peas, beans, lentils, seeds and nuts. All these foods are rich in nutrients and filled with fiber, protein, protective antioxidants, B vitamins, essential fatty acids and minerals.

Serving sizes are as follows: four ounces of tempeh of tofu, half a cup of cooked beans, one ounce of seeds or nuts, one cup of soy milk and two tablespoons of seed or nut butter.

Grains

- Four to six serving daily

Whole grains equip your body with minerals, B vitamins, antioxidants, fiber and protein. They are far healthier than their refined counterparts, as the process of refinement removes a lot of the nutrients. Additionally, intact or uncut whole grains like oats, rice, quinoa (which is actually a seed that is used like a grain) and millet are far superior in nutritional value than flours made from whole grains, flaked or puffed whole grains.

Serving sizes are: one bread slice, one-ounce cereal and half a cup of cooked grain. This is only a guideline as this group of foods is quite flexible as far as serving sizes are concerned and you may vary your intake according to your own energy needs.

Vegetables

- Four or more serving daily.

You should try to eat a large variety of vegetables of all colors each day. This will provide you with an array of nutrients.

A serving of veggies would be one cup of raw, half a cup of cooked or half a cup of vegetable juice. It is almost impossible to consume too much of this food group, particularly the leafy greens rich in calcium.

Fruits

- Two or more servings daily.

Most of the fruits are rich in vitamin C, especially berries and citrus fruits, and fiber and antioxidants are present in all of them. Whole fruits are more beneficial than juices; they also contain more fiber.

A fruit serving would be: a medium sized piece, a quarter cup of dried or one cup of sliced fruit and a quarter cup of fruit juice.

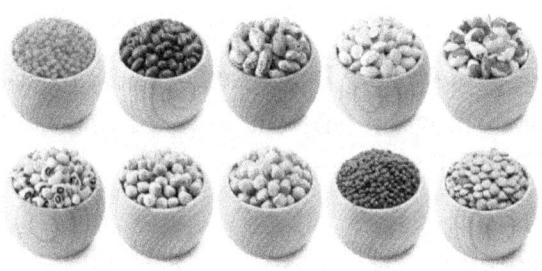

Just How Healthy Can a Vegan Diet Be?

In 2009 the Dietetic Association of America published a paper on the different vegetarian diets in which they state that a vegan diet is quite adequate as far as nutrition is concerned and that it is a healthy diet. They went on to say that these diets may present health benefits for the treatment and prevention of a number of diseases. A well-balanced vegan diet will help to decrease the occurrence of cancer, heart diseases, diabetes and obesity.

Pay attention to these nutrients

Just like everybody else, regardless of which diet they are following, vegans have to be vigilant and make sure they get all the necessary nutrients their bodies need to stay healthy. The most important ones to look out for are the omega three fatty acids, and vitamins D and B12.

- Vitamin B12 assists the body in the proper formation of the red blood cells, with the body's neurological functions and with its DNA synthesis. This vitamin is made by certain kinds of bacteria encountered in nature. We get this vitamin from the plants we eat, but because they vary greatly in the amount of bacteria they contain and because we tend to scrub our food clean, we should not totally rely on this source for our vitamin B12 needs. Therefore, we have to consume fortified foods or take supplements. You can use any vegan source of two thousand micrograms weekly as supplement or else ten to one hundred micrograms daily. If you are not a fan of supplements, make sure to consume three or more servings daily of fortified food. These foods include nondairy milks, beverage mixes, breakfast cereals, nutritional yeast formula for vegetarian support (Red Star) or meal replacement or stand-in bars.

- Vitamin D, also called our sunshine vitamin, is manufactured by our skin from the sun's ultraviolet rays. It is a hormone and plays a vital role in the health of our bones. Additionally, it supports immune and normal neuromuscular function. A regular, adequate intake of this vitamin will prevent or at least lower your risk of certain cancers, osteoporosis as well as various chronic diseases.

- Deficient levels of Vitamin D are a health concern in the populations of many countries all around the world. You may not realize it but it is definitely not that easy to get enough of this vitamin. Many factors can influence our skin's ability to manufacture the hormone from the rays of the sun, like skin pigmentation, clothing, the seasons, sunscreen, latitude and air pollution, amongst others. Furthermore, it is encountered in very few foods. That is why everyone, including vegans, must make sure they get ample doses of vitamin D. Recent research found that even the recommended allowance might not be sufficient for a lot of people. The suggestion is to take one to two thousand IU or international units daily. This will of course depend on the various needs of different individuals.

Vitamin D supplements come in the following three forms: ergocalciferol (Vegan D2) which is either made from yeast or is a synthetic product, vegan D3 made from lichen, or cholecalciferol (D3 non-vegan) which is made from lanolin that is found in the wool of sheep.

- Omega three fatty acids are essential for the optimal functioning of our brains, the health status of our hearts and infant and child development. ALA (alpha linolenic acid) is one of these fatty acids which in part convert to EPA and DHA in our bodies. It can be found in a number of edible plants like hemp and flax products, walnuts, green leafy veggies and canola oil. Two to four grams of this ALA should be consumed daily.

The following is an indication of serving sizes and the amount in grams of ALA it contains:
- Two cups of mixed green - 0.2
- Half a cup of firm tofu – 0.7
- One tablespoon of canola oil – 1.6
- A quarter cup of walnuts – 2.7
- Two tablespoons of ground flaxseed – 3.8
- Two tablespoons of whole flaxseed – 5.2
- One tablespoon of flaxseed oil – 8.0

How about protein?

We all know that protein helps to build healthy bones and muscle, it repairs tissue, keeps our immune system healthy and lots more. Between ten and twenty percent of the calories in plant foods like veggies, grains and legumes come from protein but we humans only need between ten and fifteen percent of these kind of calories; it is not difficult to meet the necessary requirements by eating a good variety of plant foods. There is no need to 'complement' our plant proteins because our bodies store the amino acids necessary to manufacture complete proteins from our meals during the day.

Gender and age will determine your recommended allowance for protein and other factors like pregnancy, health status and activity levels will also play a role. If you want a general idea of your required daily intake of protein in grams, multiply your weight (measured in pounds) by 0.36. For example, an adult weighing one hundred and fifty pounds will need around fifty-five grams.

The following is an example of a meal plan which will give you seventy-seven grams protein, more than most people need.

Breakfast:
- Oatmeal, one and a half cups – 9g, plus walnuts 1oz – 4g, plus cinnamon
- Small banana – one g

Lunch:
- 3 Bean chili, one and a half cups – 16g
- Jalapeno cornbread, 1 piece with maple spread – 2g
- Vegetable salad 2 cups – 4g

Dinner:
- Sweet potato, bok choy, onion, broccoli stir-fried, 2 cups – 5g
- Orange sesame baked tofu 4oz – 7g
- Brown rice 2 cups – 9g

Snacks:

- Peanut butter 2tbsp – 8g and crackers, whole grain – 3g
- Fruit – 1g
- Trail mix 2oz – 8g

How about calcium?

In the plant kingdom, calcium is found in abundance in nature. Therefore, whole plant foods can fulfil all our needs in this regard. Otherwise foods that are calcium fortified can be consumed. An adult need around one thousand mg daily, but it will vary according to which stage you have reached in your lifecycle. Select several foods rich in calcium from every group to include in your diet daily. Plants high in calcium content are figs, green leafy veggies, sesame, almonds, other nuts, calcium tofu, beans, non-dairy yoghurt, breakfast cereals, soy products and fruit juice (all fortified).

The following is a list of serving sizes and the amount of calcium in mg they contain:
- Half a cup of calcium set tofu – between 140 and 420

- One cup of soy milk, fortified - between 200 and 370
- One cup collard greens, cooked – between 270 and 360
- Orange juice, fortified – between 300 and 350
- One cup of soy yoghurt – between 150 and 350
- One cup of cooked amaranth - 275
- Half a bunch of cooked broccoli rabe or Rapini – 260
- Two tablespoons of unhulled sesame seeds – 175
- One tablespoon of blackstrap molasses – between 80 and 170
- One cup of cooked navy beans – 160
- One cup of cooked bok choy – 110
- One ounce of almonds – 70

Chapter 4 How to Make the Transition to Veganism

After reading the first three chapters, you have come to the conclusion that it will be to your benefit to change to a vegan life style. But now, how to go about it? It might seem a daunting task at the moment, but changing your diet is in actual fact not that scary at all. The secret is taking 'baby steps'. Focus on one small adjustment, then the next and very soon the progression will become natural. As long as you make the changes at your individual pace, and follow a method suitable to your needs, it will be much easier than you imagined. I will now provide you with a few pointers and ideas to assist you with this process but remember to adjust them to fit your distinct needs.

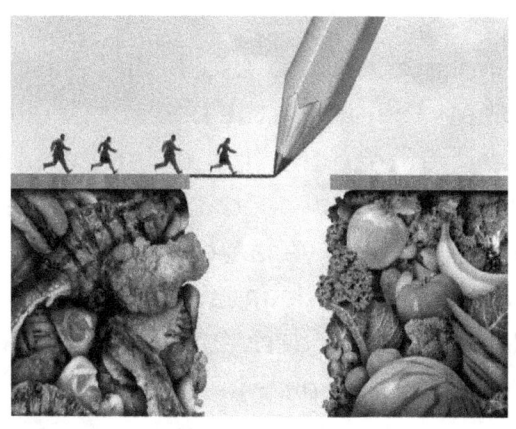

Gather Enough Information

Do not start the transition before you are completely informed and confident that you know and understand veganism thoroughly. This will prevent doubts and you will feel much more prepared for the change in the lifestyle you are embarking on.

- Read about the many benefits of veganism and learn about the costs and practices behind the manufacturing of all kinds of animal-derived products. You have to determine why it is that you want to become a vegan; this will be your driving force.

- Find out how to use a diet based on plants to nourish the body optimally.
- Start to read the lists of ingredients on products. You need to know whether products are vegan or not. Make sure you are knowledgeable about all the lesser known derivatives from animals which may appear in ingredients.
- Inspect your local store for their vegan products and locate the vegan restaurants and specialty stores around your area.
- Watch, read a lot of research and learn. Fish for information and opinions in vegan books, documentaries, websites, magazines, forums, blogs and talk to veteran vegans. There is a wealth of information and insights out there which can be invaluable to make you feel confident about your transition.

Add to Your Existing Diet Before Subtracting from It

- Explore the preparation, uses and storage of ingredients like whole grains,

nuts, legumes, beans, tofu and seeds and start incorporating them into your meals. Make sure you are familiar enough with these items.
- Collect vegan recipes and begin experimenting with them to find out what appeals to you.
- Swap your milk for an alternative which is non-dairy like soy or almond.

Most people find this an easy enough switch to make, but since there are so many options you have to find your own favorites.

Seek and Keep in Mind Your Strongest Motivation for The Change

To adopt a vegan diet and lifestyle is very different from simply going on some new diet. People on diets often cheat or stray from their diet plan but veganism is a different ball-game altogether. Veganism is more than a diet; it is a new way of looking at things and once you have made the commitment you do not want to easily wander from it again.

Hence, it is very important that you are familiar with the health benefits and the adverse effects all animal products can have on the environment, your health and humanity as a whole. Once you realize this, you will not normally want to go back to your old lifestyle again.

Keep Up Your Positive Attitude
Concentrate on all the delicious new foods you are trying out instead of thinking about those that you are discarding from your diet. It will be a pleasant surprise to find just how numerous your options actually are. You may find that lots of your old favorites come in a vegan version already and there are hundreds of interesting international dishes suitable for a vegan diet. You can even turn your old favorites into vegan friendly dishes yourself. So, keep the excitement going and focus on your new culinary adventure.

Start to Plan Your Transition

Now you have to really get down to business and decide which way of going vegan will work the best for your needs. Here are some of the most common options:

From vegetarian to vegan

- Change to a vegetarian diet and then progress into veganism. This can be done all at once in one leap or you can cut out eggs and dairy one by one.

From omnivore to veganism, a slow transition

- Cut out the animal products in your diet slowly. Start with those ones that are easy and leave the more difficult options for last.

Gradually reduce intake of animal product

As you slowly decrease your intake of the animal products, simultaneously increase your consumption of plant foods. Continue this process until all products coming from animals have been eliminated.

Vegan all out

- Banish all ingredients derived from animals from your diet and incorporate beans, whole grains, tofu, seeds, nuts and legumes in all your meals.
- Swap every single non-vegan ingredient for the vegan alternative. People often find that eating vegan hot dogs, hamburgers, cheeses and deli slices is a tremendous help in the transition when they decide to banish all animal products from their diet immediately.

Guidelines and Ideas for Different Approaches

Now I want to provide you with a few guidelines and ideas for each of the above-mentioned approaches. Select the one which appeals most to you personally and adapt it to suit you.

From vegetarian to vegan

- Start by removing meat products from your diet; that includes poultry and fish. Do not eat more dairy and eggs to replace the meat; rather increase your intake of protein sources which are plant based.
- Read the ingredients labels carefully and avoid everything which contains rennet, gelatin and other products from animals, excluding eggs and dairy.
- Maybe you have already done so, but remember to incorporate more beans, whole grains, tofu, seeds, nuts and legumes into your meals.
- As soon as you are comfortable to proceed, begin to phase out eggs, dairy and honey. Take it slowly; there is no time restriction and tackle the food groups one by one, at your own pace.

From omnivore to veganism, a slow transition

- Start by eliminating your least desired animal products.

- Now incorporate more beans, whole grains, seeds, tofu, legumes and nuts while you eliminate more animal products, especially the ones you will not really miss.
- You can either gradually begin to exclude one food or food group or to lessen your intake of animal products.
- Focus on barrier foods only after you are completely comfortable and happy with all of the other changes you have made towards your new diet.
- Read the ingredient lists; start by avoiding those animal products least obvious and noticeable one by one. Otherwise you may decide to just overlook them for now and start by removing the more obvious animal derived products like seafood, meat, eggs, dairy products etc. Once you have achieved this, move on to the elimination of less obvious products.

Go vegan all out

Maybe you are one of those brave people who always jump right in. Well, then why wait? Just keep on educating yourself to be one hundred percent prepared for the jump. Make sure you learn about the following:

- How to get the optimum nutrition on your vegan diet
- How do I know whether something is vegan?
- How do I draw up a healthy, well-balanced grocery list for vegans?
- Veganism on a budget
- FAQ for beginner vegans

I have already mentioned that some people take the option of counting on vegan substitutes of their old favorites in the beginning. These are usually protein rich, fortified with minerals and vitamins, easy and quick to prepare, familiar and delicious. I must point out though that some of the vegan hot dogs, veggie burgers, deli slices and others are highly processed. Try to gradually lessen the consumption of these easy options as you become more adjusted to your new lifestyle. They may be consumed in moderation, at times, but must never be the main source for minerals, protein and vitamins in your diet.

Veganism is a lifestyle of compassion, not merely a diet. The most challenging part of veganism is the transition; therefore, I have given you some guidelines to follow. These however are only as far as your diet is concerned. You should follow this up by also eliminating the use of all other items derived from animals like clothing, shoes, make-up and household items.

Food Barriers and The Idea of All or Nothing

It is perfectly normal to fear the cravings for your favorite foods and the thought of having to give them up when you turn vegan. You, like everyone before you, will face your own difficulties but they need not be unbreakable barriers. The majority of people make the switch to veganism for ethical reasons and not because of their enjoyment of the taste of animal derived foods. You may find it strange but it is true that there are many vegans who actually love cheese.

Many people discard the notion of becoming a vegan out of fear; they can think only about that one kind of food they will miss so much. Others embark on the journey, but throw in the towel for the same reason. This mostly happens when people have tried to jump into veganism without proper preparation or otherwise proceed too quickly. To make it sustainable you have to go at your own pace; one that you are comfortable with.

The following are a few methods for dealing with food barriers effectively:
- Acquaint yourself with practices involved in the production of your favored foods.
- Investigate the details of this food production. Often this will be enough to convince you of the reasonableness of your decision to discard this particular food.

- Banish all your barrier foods from your diet in one shot. Most of the time these cravings are only felt for a few weeks after which they subside.
- Slowly replace your favorites with their vegan alternatives. Some food items need more time to get used to like yoghurt and cheese, so do not be in a hurry to substitute them; rather go without them in the meantime.
- You will have to experiment with all the various options to find out which of the products you enjoy most and also try out different ways of preparing them. Through trial and error, you will soon establish which ones are your favorites.

Focus on barrier foods last

If you are eager to adopt veganism but dread the notion of giving up one specific food and fear you will not be able to do so, go ahead with the transition but leave that specific food until last. Once you tackle it, do so very slowly and in a controlled manner. Take a couple of weeks, even longer if necessary. By now, you have accomplished the bulk of the transition process and will probably find that it is much easier to exclude your old highly-liked food item than you had anticipated.

Maybe that barrier food is a hurdle that you simply cannot clear and it is preventing you from achieving a hundred percent vegan lifestyle. Do not despair! Just do not allow that to stand in your way of minimizing your consumption of animal derived products as far as possible. Give up as much as you find possible and occasionally allow yourself an exception like a holiday food, favorite restaurant or food.

Adopting a one hundred percent vegan lifestyle is what you should strive for, and see it as the ultimate goal. Still, it would be plain silly to give up your efforts entirely only because you cannot part with cheese or bacon. Do not label or define yourself by the diet you are following; it would be deconstructive and this 'everything or nothing' approach will not do you any good. If you are only capable of living a vegan life by allowing a certain measure of flexibility, then that is what you must do. This outlook will help to make veganism a less daunting idea and help others to find it more approachable.

Helpful Reminders and Hints

Remember that every tiny bit counts. Regardless of whether you turn vegetarian or vegan or just decide to reduce your intake of animal derived foods, you are on the right track. Do not fall for the idea of a label to define you. You are not your diet; you are much more than that.

Becoming a vegan is not as difficult as most people think, but there are skills involved to achieve success, certain learning curves to follow. So, never become overwhelmed, take all the time you need and expect a few mistakes on the way. You will learn from these mishaps and can then move on.

Chapter 5 How to Budget for a Vegan Lifestyle

Regardless of your income, it definitely is possible to tailor your vegan lifestyle to fit your budget. The myth that veganism is costly is totally unfounded. Truth be told, the opposite is true; vegan diets can accommodate any budgetary restrictions. The foods that make up the staples of typical vegan diets are all very affordable, for example grains, seeds, beans and legumes. It is possible to make lots of different delicious vegan meals without over-spending. Broth based or creamy soups, vegetable curries on tofu or rice, stir-fried veggies, salads, pasta dishes, sandwiches and bean and vegetable chilies are just a few of the affordable and tasty vegan meals which will not cost you an arm and a leg.

If your shift to veganism has inspired you to eat healthier meals, you may be tempted to try those "super foods" that are available. It is a wonderful idea, but these pricy foods are surely not your only choice for a balanced and healthy vegan diet. In this chapter, I will give you some ideas that will help you to save a lot of money while still following your healthy new dietary plan.

Always Compare Prices

In general, grocery stores will display unit prices for their items, but often they also show the cost in weight for certain products. Do not be misled by unit prices; compare the prices of different sized packaging by using their cost in weight. You will find that the cheaper packet may turn out the more expensive one by weight. Also compare prices between different brands for the same item.

Frozen versus fresh

If you love smoothies, add lots of fruit to your oatmeal or use fruit in your baking, then you should consider buying the frozen product. Be careful when you compare the prices though, since frozen fruit are sometimes more costly than the fresh produce. If your store has a special on fresh fruit, buy sufficiently and then freeze it yourself. It works well with bananas, berries and other kinds of fruit used in smoothies. You probably are not aware that frozen fruit are higher in nutritional value than the fresh produce because they are frozen right at their peak ripeness. They also do not lose any nutrients due to transport time like their fresh counterparts on their way to the grocery store. And no nutrients are lost during the process of freezing.

Bulk versus packaged

A wonderful way to save your hard-earned money is to buy items in bulk, especially those that come in smaller packages and are used in small amounts. Large packages are often cheaper by weight. Great foods to get in bulk include:
- Herbs and spices
- Seeds and nuts
- Grains

- Flours
- Snack items
- Dried fruit (ensure they are packaged almost airtight and not dried out too much)
- Items new to you that are more expensive (try them out before you purchase or you may end up with a lot of something you do not actually like).

Organic versus non-organic

Normally organic food items are more expensive so it is entirely your choice whether you buy them or not. Even if you are not really interested in organic produce, do check that section out from time to time. You may find something there on sale that actually works out cheaper than the one you generally buy.

Brand name versus generic brand

Always watch out for the generic brands when you go shopping; they are usually cheaper and can save you a lot of money in the long run. Items to look out for are:

- Pasta
- Baking supplies like baking powder, salt, baking soda, corn starch, flours etc.
- Oatmeal
- Seeds and nuts
- Dried fruit
- Rice

Compare different grocery stores

You can easily compare the prices of all the grocery stores in your area online and only then write down your grocery shopping list accordingly. If you are lucky enough to have a few stores located close to home or around your workplace, consider purchasing from all of them when they have sales. This may take more time, but you will go home with more dollars in your pocket than you budgeted for. The best time for sales shopping is early in the morning to ensure you still get the best choices before everything has been sold out.

Consider membership at a good wholesaler

It is really worth your while to get a membership card at a good wholesale store, even if you have a small family or live alone. Before you purchase your membership though, visit the store with a friend or acquaintance who is already a member to see what they have on their shelves and to decide whether it will suit your needs. When shopping for a smaller number of people, do not be tempted to buy too much; focus on non-perishable items and check the sell-by dates carefully.

This will prevent wastage. Foods to buy at a wholesaler include:
- Grains
- Frozen vegetables and fruit
- Cooking oils
- Cereals like granola, oatmeal etc.
- Bread (extras can be frozen)
- Seeds and nuts
- Nut butters
- Baking supplies

- Crackers, protein bars, chips and other vegan snacks
- Hummus

Search for cheaper options of super foods and vegan specialty foods items

Treat yourself from time to time on one of these fancier items, especially after you have saved on your budget by buying in bulk or at a sale. Try something new for fun.

Markdowns in grocery stores

Always visit the marked-down sections of your grocery stores to take advantage of their twenty-five and fifty percent markdowns. Many stores actually do their cost lowering later in the afternoon before closing, while others do it just before opening, so find out when it will take place to enable you to be there at the right time and get the best produce.

If you live in a rural area or a city with a small vegan or vegetarian community, you may find the vegan substitutes and specialty foods more expensive. Fortunately, the turn-over rate will be slower and there will be more opportunities for special offers and clearance sales. Check out the dates on the items you are interested in and return a day or two before the sell-by date. You can find out from the manager how long before they reach their 'best before' day they will be marked down so that you can visit the store then.

Wholesalers

Like I have mentioned above, you should consider buying a membership card for a wholesaler. You will save a lot on items such as convenience foods, vegan bars, snack foods, nut butters, hemp hearts and chia seeds, as well as other super foods.

Online retailers

Lots of great discounts and deals are to be found online, so do your research and utilize these options. Sites to check out are iHerb and Better Health Store, especially for supplements, specialty foods and items for personal care. Coupon codes, sales and referrals are great for even cheaper deals.

Prepare and Cook Your Own Food

Prepare your convenience meals at home
We all know that pre-packaged meals and foods work out more expensively than home cooked food. So, you can actually save lots of money by preparing and cooking your own snacks and meals. Are you often in a situation that you run out of time and have to buy convenience food? Consider purchasing a well-insulated lunch box of the right size to pack your home-made snacks and lunches in. You can even utilize the reusable bag you use for your groceries instead of buying an expensive new lunch box. Freeze a water bottle to keep your meal cool until you consume it. Afterwards you will also be able to enjoy the cold water to quench your thirst. With

a little planning, you can cut down on food expenses substantially.

Concentrate on whole foods for your diet

Fortunately for vegans, the bulk of their staples are really affordable, like frozen and fresh fruit and veggies in season, beans, whole grains, nuts, tofu and legumes. Keep all the tips above in mind when you do your shopping to guarantee you purchase at the lowest prices possible.

- Vegetables and fruit: Select those items that are in season or on sale. If you find a good deal, stock up; you can freeze what you do not use immediately. Keep your eyes peeled for markdowns and sales amongst the frozen items too.

- Grains: Look out for store brands as well as economy sized boxes and bags of whole wheat pastas and brown rice. When purchasing baked goods, search for sales, good deals and markdowns. Stock up, portion and freeze; by only taking out what you will use the following day you will prevent wastage and save money. Also store your wraps, bread, bagels, English muffins etc. in your freezer and defrost only what you will need daily. If you follow this simple rule, nothing will go to waste.

- Legumes and beans: These items are usually quite affordable. Try to use dried beans and keep the more expensive canned products only for convenience. Although they are costlier, they are still a viable option, but remember when you buy canned foods, always pick the ones with the lowest amount of sodium. Fresh tofu is another budget-friendly food and if you find it amongst the sale items buy in bulk since it can be frozen successfully. Its texture becomes a bit chewier and works wonderfully when you use it to substitute the ground beef used in pasta or chili recipes.

- Seeds and nuts: Buy these items in bulk and package it according to your needs.

Always check the expiry date to make sure you do not buy more than you can use; you will save money by purchasing the largest bag available so you do not want to waste money by wasting food you cannot consume in time. Remember that seeds and nuts can also be frozen.

- Avoid the vegan substitutes: Vegan cheeses and meat substitutes are often the same price as their medium quality non-vegan equivalents.

- If you compare their volumes, you will find that the substitutes are more expensive. Watch out for discounts and sales; that is the time to invest in these kinds of foods. If appropriate, freeze them or otherwise use them without too long a delay. Find a good recipe and make vegan burgers yourself; they are more nutritious, cheaper and fresher than most veggie burgers you can buy in the store.

Make the Most of Your Trip to the Stores

Staples stock-up

If you find food items which you know you will consume before they expire, buy in volume. Look out for the dates on packages. If a food item is a good buy, purchase more than one packet if the expiry date allows it. Non-dairy milks that can be kept on the shelf are a great example since they have an expiry date of one month if not opened.

Schedule your shopping trips

Work out a schedule which suits your needs and then stick to that schedule. If you decide to shop for groceries every seven days, plan to buy just enough lest you have wastage. Save all your receipts to keep track of what and how much you buy during every shopping trip. Doing it this way, you will not run out or overstock on any items. Very soon you will know exactly which items to eliminate or reduce in quantity during your shopping and which to add to your list.

Build Your Own Budget List for Groceries

A vegan diet has many benefits and one of these is the fact that it is not necessary to have to purchase so many fancy ingredients and 'super foods'. On an affordable budget you can enjoy delicious, healthy meals; all it takes is a little dedication and planning. Work out your budget for food spending and then do not over-step that mark. I find that it helps to tally in my head as I go along during my shopping trip to ensure I do not end up at spending double my budget for the week.

The tips mentioned above should keep you on the right track. Stay with the staples like beans, whole grains, frozen and fresh veggies and fruit, tofu, seeds, nuts and legumes. You will soon find building your personal budget list for the groceries you need a breeze.

What types of foods and meals can be prepared on a budget?
- Salads
- Pasta dishes
- Stir-fries
- Wraps and sandwiches
- Chili
- Soups
- Burrito bowls
- Peanut butter and apples
- Banana sandwiches with peanut butter
- Vegetables and hummus
- Smoothies
- Baked fries
- Baked potatoes
- Oatmeal with toppings
- Pancakes
- And lots more!

Chapter 6 Frequently Asked Questions

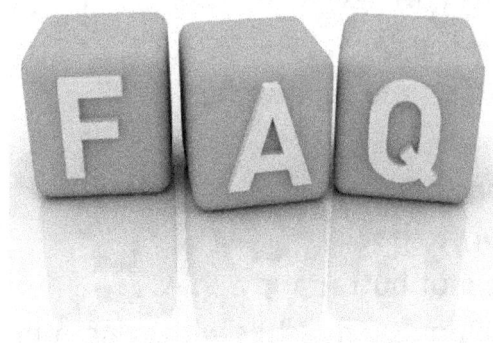

1.Is it difficult to become a vegan?

You might find it hard if you go about it the wrong way. If you attempt to make the change too quickly and endeavor to achieve a very high standard right from the start, you may encounter difficulties. It is important to make the changes at a pace that will suit you. Also make the changes in your lifestyle in a way that leaves you feeling comfortable. Ideally you may want to eliminate animal products from your diet completely, but in the meantime, any cutback will put you on the way towards that goal. Adopting a vegan lifestyle takes time and is a continuous process. Everyone will go about it at his or her own pace so remember that each step you take towards veganism is a positive one.

Place your focus on abstaining from all those products that animals are slaughtered and bred for. Products derived from animals will be with us until the demand for dairy products and primary meat ceases. As far as items with smaller amounts of animal by-products are concerned, every vegan will have to make his or her own decision and decide what they find acceptable or not. I will give you an example: You may avoid bread baked with whey when you do your shopping but at a dinner party you may eat bread without concerning yourself with its ingredients. These kinds of compromises may actually encourage others to pursue a vegan diet, because it makes them realize that it really is not that hard to live as a vegan.

2. Is it expensive to be a vegan?

It is true that some of the substitutes for dairy and meat can be pricy, but there are many products for vegans which are quite inexpensive, like oatmeal, bagels, peanut butter, pasta, bread, tortillas, tomato sauce, beans, potatoes, rice, as well as common produce. The vegan (and vegetarian) market is growing fast and this allows for more competition and innovation with increasing availability of vegan products which in turn drive costs down.

3. Are 99% vegan foods acceptable?

Sometimes you will find products on the shelve with a vegan label but with another one stating that it is ninety-nine percent dairy free. Usually this means that these products were made using machines or equipment that are also used for the productions of dairy products. Therefore, there may be lingering traces of dairy found on the machines. Some people are severely allergic to dairy; thus, the manufacturer cannot take the chance to claim that its products are one hundred percent free of dairy traces. The only alternative is to clean the machinery with steam before making their carob chips, and this will not contribute to the advancement of veganism's cause because no animals are being exploited in this process. The contrary is true; the cost of these chips will increase and be less tempting to vegan customers and general consumers.

4.Which are the hidden animal ingredients?

The list is long so it is recommended that the prospective vegan concentrates on the more obvious ingredients than try to read every single piece of information and just become bogged down and frustrated. Do not be burdened with too much detail while missing the whole point of true veganism.

5. What is the feeling about silk and honey?

Every person has his own definition of veganism. Insects are considered as animals so all products derived from them like silk and honey are generally not appropriate for vegans. Having said that, I have to point out that there are many vegans who have no objection to products derived from insects because they believe insects are not conscious of any pain. It really depends on the individual since the debate is an ongoing one. If your houseguest is a vegan or you are labelling food suitable for vegans, better be safe than sorry and avoid insect products like honey.

6. How do I cope with food allergies?

If you are allergic to wheat or suffer from gluten intolerance, do not fear. There are many alternatives for grain which are healthy and suitable for a vegan. In actual fact, products like millet and quinoa are far superior in nutritional value than wheat.

Previously products like crackers and bread were made only with varieties of wheat but these are now freely available without gluten and wheat. Even an allergy for soy is not a problem anymore; it is only one of the numerous foods suitable for vegans. Soy based alternatives for meat should in this instance be substituted for wheat or nut based varieties like seitan. Very few individuals are intolerant to all seeds and nuts, so find out exactly which ones you are allergic to and stay clear of those. Many substitutes are suitable for use in recipes as well as foods like trail mixes, seed and nut butters and granola.

7.I felt unhealthy on my vegan diet. What went wrong?

Any dietary changes may affect your digestion and health, making you feel fatigued or prone to cravings. When you replace the junk food with plant food and eliminate some animal products from your diet, your body might start to complain. Any major dietary change will cause some bodily discomfort for a while, especially if you increase your fiber intake drastically over a short time period. This should be temporary so if the symptoms persist for longer than three days, consult your doctor to eliminate any accidental health conditions.

Even the best intentions to change to a vegan diet may backfire if your diet does not turn out to be well balanced. A common mistake many first-time vegans make is to eat fewer calories than is necessary. Vegan diets are usually voluminous, even more so when you concentrate on fresh raw fruit and vegetables; your plate must be filled and overflowing with food. But you still might not be getting enough calories and this will leave you feeling tired, irritable and hungry.

8. Is it at all possible to eat too much?

Too much of any good thing is not good any more. So, yes, it is definitely possible to consume too much of a food. Vegans tend to consume a lot of processed soy because they like the texture and flavors which mimic that of dairy and meat. If your intake of soy is too high, it means that it replaces some other foods and thus the balance of your diet is compromised. A daily intake of no more than two servings of processed soy is acceptable. Soy products that are less processed or fermented like edamame, tempeh, miso, fortified soymilk from organic beans and tofu are the healthiest option.

8. Is it at all possible to eat too much?

Too much of any good thing is not good any more. So, yes, it is definitely possible to consume too much of a food. Vegans tend to consume a lot of processed soy because they like the texture and flavors which mimic that of dairy and meat. If your intake of soy is too high, it means that it replaces some other foods and thus the balance of your diet is compromised. A daily intake of no more than two servings of processed soy is acceptable. Soy products that are less processed or fermented like edamame, tempeh, miso, fortified soymilk from organic beans and tofu are the healthiest option.

Conclusion

If you had any doubts in the beginning, I am sure you are now more convinced that a vegan diet and lifestyle may be the option for you and everyone else for that matter. By now you know just how easy it really is to make these changes to your diet and how to go about it in a practical way that you feel comfortable with. You will enter into this new lifestyle gradually and at a pace which will not leave you feeling overwhelmed. You have been given all the information to ensure that your new diet is a well-balanced one which contains all the nutrients your body needs. Your health will improve; you will sleep better and not gain unnecessary weight because your body is getting the best nutrition possible to function optimally.

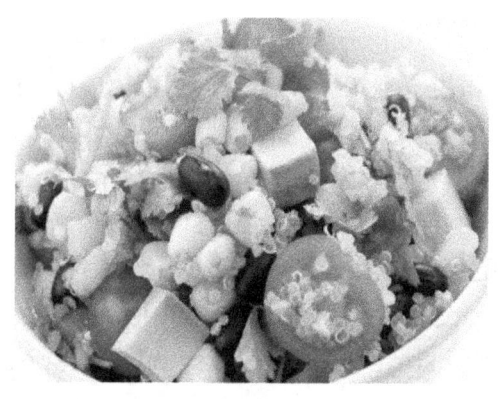

You will discover new foods and recipes that you have never knew existed and embark on a completely new culinary journey. Including lots of raw vegetables and fruit into your diet will leave you with extra time on your hands because there will be less cooking required. You can still go to restaurants since many of them have caught on and now offer a variety of delicious vegan dishes. Shopping for your vegan food is not a problem either; it is readily available in supermarkets and health stores. And you will benefit financially too, since the staples that make up a vegan diet are not costly and can often be bought in bulk.

Not only will your health improve, you will make your contribution to the welfare of our animals and help to eliminate the raising and slaughtering of farm stock without regard for their suffering. Animals are sentient beings and experience emotions like pain, anxiety, loneliness and fear and should be treated with respect.

Lastly, when you switch to a vegan lifestyle you will know that you are doing your little bit to save our planet, not only for your children but for future generations.

About the Author

Allen Dial is author of several cookbooks on Vegan diet. He has written research papers on the topic and currently lives in California.

www.ingramcontent.com/pod-product-compliance
Lightning Source LLC
LaVergne TN
LVHW011943070526
838202LV00054B/4781